ABORIGINAL AND TORRES STRAIT ISLANDER PEOPLES' HEALTHCARE

BRETT BILES AND JESSICA BILES

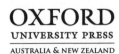

OXFORD
UNIVERSITY PRESS
AUSTRALIA & NEW ZEALAND

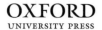

Oxford University Press is a department of the University of Oxford.
It furthers the University's objective of excellence in research,
scholarship, and education by publishing worldwide. Oxford is a registered
trademark of Oxford University Press in the UK and in certain other
countries.

Published in Australia by
Oxford University Press
8/737 Bourke Street, Docklands Victoria 3008, Australia

 A catalogue record for this
book is available from the
National Library of Australia

ISBN 9780190311445

Reproduction and communication for educational purposes
The Australian Copyright Act 1968 (the Act) allows educational
institutions that are covered by remuneration arrangements
with Copyright Agency to reproduce and communicate certain
material for educational purposes. For more information,
see copyright.com.au.

Edited by Pete Cruttenden
Typeset by Newgen KnowledgeWorksPvt. Ltd., Chennai, India
Indexed by Jeanne Rudd
Printed in China by Leo Paper Products Ltd

Links to third party websites are provided by Oxford in good faith and for information only.

*Oxford disclaims any responsibility for the materials contained in any third party website
referenced in this work.*

Dedication

For Norman Dulvarie

CONTENTS

PART 1: FRAMEWORKS FOR HEALTH AND COMPETENCE

PART 2: CONTEXTS OF HEALTHCARE

OXFORD UNIVERSITY PRESS

LIST OF FIGURES AND TABLES

FIGURES

TABLES

LIST OF CASE STUDIES

OXFORD UNIVERSITY PRESS

FOREWORD

It is with respect, passion and wisdom that I provide the foreword for this book.

This book is a valuable resource for nursing and allied health professionals who are currently studying or working in the healthcare environment. Especially to those clinicians that are delivering health services to Aboriginal and Torres Strait Islander peoples across the maze of health services systems.

We are the oldest continuing culture in the world and this highlights that we have had systems in place that are sustainable and focus on holistic practices. We need mainstream health services to be responsive to the needs of Aboriginal and Torres Strait Islander peoples and to acknowledge that we come with over 40,000 years of lived experience that has been passed down from generation to generation.

This textbook is written from a strengths-based approach which highlights the strength and resilience of Aboriginal and Torres Strait Islander peoples and our strong connection to land and culture. This book underpins the holistic approach to healthcare and its interconnectedness within the wider healthcare systems.

In addition, this book has relied on the Aboriginal Australian cultural competency framework throughout the content. For some it has been a journey of challenges that have been presented by the establishment of policies that have been thrust upon us over time. It requires self-reflection on our beliefs, attitudes and values and then to consider how these may influence, change or enhance the care we provide to our clients without bias. I strongly encourage you to reflect on who you are as a person and how your beliefs and attitudes can enhance or inhibit health outcomes for your clients.

We as Aboriginal and Torres Strait Islander peoples are diverse and have the right to self-determination to enhance our health and wellbeing outcomes. The 'one size fits all' approach to improve health outcomes has been proven not to work. However, if we learn to listen from our elders and communities regarding the local health needs, we will be in a better position to provide health services that will meet those needs. The answer begins with understanding the differences in culture. Aboriginal and non-Aboriginal health workers working together through robust partnerships and respecting each other's qualities will provide a healthy platform toward achieving better health outcomes for Aboriginal and Torres Strait Islander people.

A key feature of this book is the accompanying audio-visual components which allow you to hear and see the lived experiences of Aboriginal people as we navigate through the health systems of this land.

I recommend this book to all health professionals. Remember that Aboriginal Australian cultural competence is a lifelong journey that does not stop.

LaVerne Bellear
Chief Executive Officer, Redfern Aboriginal Medical Service

FROM THE EDITORS

As editors we have worked together not only to facilitate the writing collaboration but also to develop the overall philosophical standpoint of the text. Our personal influences as editors have also contributed to the direction of the writing.

We are married and have two daughters, Stella and Audrey. Our personal experiences both as individuals and as a family have influenced our sense of being in the world and thus the development and influence of this textbook. After many years teaching Aboriginal and Torres Strait Islander peoples' health in the fields of education and healthcare, it has become clear that the pedagogical focus of teaching and learning was often on the deficit model. For example, teaching and learning in the field has often concentrated on the health disparity compared with non-Indigenous people, and how health professionals can contribute to Aboriginal and Torres Strait Islander peoples' wellness. We have tried to shift the focus in this text by using the philosophy of Indigenous Australian cultural competence, where the onus of responsibility is not on the patient but instead on the clinician—how the clinician can adapt to meet the needs of the client, rather than how can the client must adapt to meet the needs of the health professional. Coupled with personal experiences raising two girls, we both felt that there was much to learn from history, a need to reconsider our thinking in working collaboratively with clients, and a need to celebrate successes. In the world we live in, we hear too frequently about tragedy, and while this is appropriate, it displays unequivocal bias when the celebration of successes is ignored.

We have both experienced challenges within our respective professions and at times have needed to distance ourselves from the rhetoric to be able to reflect and look forward. We are passionate that our children's generation holds the beacon of light that will see us through a new wave of thinking. Already their generation's understanding of cultural competence is far superior to our own. We can only hope this worldview will be reflected in their chosen professions as adults.

We believe that the deficit model will be slowly revoked, and instead we will see the strengths and wisdom of the oldest cultures in the world hold court. We hope that textbooks such as this will no longer be a priority or even a requirement in the future of Australian healthcare because the skills of reconciliation, cultural competence and safety will be embedded in healthcare workers' sense of being in the world.

Brett Biles and Jessica Biles

ABOUT THE AUTHORS

BRETT BILES

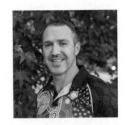

Brett Biles is a Murrawarri man from Brewarrina. He holds a Bachelor of Physiotherapy, a Masters in Indigenous Health and is currently a PhD candidate. He is currently the Director of Indigenous Health Education in the Office of Medical Education, UNSW Medicine. Prior to this he was a lecturer in Indigenous Health at the School of Nursing, Midwifery and Indigenous Health at Charles Sturt University. Brett has worked as a Lecturer in Indigenous Studies at the School of Indigenous Australian Studies and as the Academic Lead for Student Transition and Retention Program within the Faculty of Science. With a passion for education and health equality for all, Brett is an early career researcher with a keen interest in Aboriginal men and cardiovascular disease. He was named NAIDOC scholar of the year within the Albury-Wodonga community in 2018.

JESSICA BILES

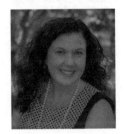

Jessica Biles holds a Bachelor of Nursing and a Masters of Health Science (Education). Her doctorate investigated Indigenous Australian cultural competence and nursing. She began her career as a nurse in metropolitan and rural hospitals in neurological, intensive care, medical and surgical, and nuclear medicine units. Jessica has also worked as a nurse in Justice Health. Jessica began work as a nurse educator in the hospital system and taught at Wodonga Institute of TAFE and Royal Melbourne Institute of Technology (Medic program), and has worked as a clinical supervisor to Bachelor of Nursing students from La Trobe University and Charles Sturt University. Jessica has held the position of lecturer within the School of Nursing, Midwifery and Indigenous Health since 2008, and is currently the Associate Head (Students) of the southern campuses. She is committed to contemporary nursing education and has worked with key nursing academics to embed and scaffold the philosophy of cultural competence across a nursing degree. She is also involved in several research projects looking at effective teaching strategies in cultural competence and evidence-based practice. Jessica is passionate about ground-up research that is driven from and by community needs.

THOMAS BRIDESON

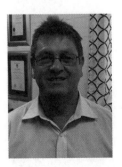

Thomas Brideson is a Kamilaroi/Gomeroi man from northwest New South Wales. For more than 25 years Tom has been actively involved in Aboriginal mental health developments, including health policy, social and emotional wellbeing, clinical mental healthcare, suicide prevention, and education. Tom has published articles regarding the Aboriginal mental health workforce and advocates for emerging degree-based professions across all health and human services. He sits on a range of mental health leadership committees and projects to improve the mental health of Aboriginal and Torres Strait Islander peoples. Tom is the state-wide coordinator of the NSW Aboriginal Mental Health Workforce Program, and chairs the National Aboriginal and Torres Strait

Islander Leadership in Mental Health Group (NATSILMH) and co-chairs the Wharerata International Indigenous Leadership Group and the National Aboriginal and Torres Strait Islander Mental Health and Suicide Prevention Advisory Group. In December 2018, Tom was appointed as a Deputy Commissioner with the NSW Mental Health Commission. Also in 2018, Tom received a Lifetime Achievement Award from IAHA for his longstanding commitment and improving the health and wellbeing of Aboriginal and Torres Strait Islander peoples.

JAMES CHARLES

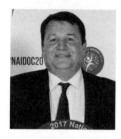

James Charles is the Coordinator of the Master of Public Health at the Institute of Koorie Education, and an academic with the School of Medicine, Deakin University. A very proud Kaurna man from the Adelaide Plains, he has lived in many different places around Australia, including Newcastle while working at the University of Newcastle and Albury while working in the Bachelor of Podiatric Medicine program at Charles Sturt University. James was one of the first Aboriginal podiatrists in Australia, the first Aboriginal person to receive a Master of Podiatry, and the first Aboriginal podiatrist to receive a PhD (Aboriginal foot health). James has volunteered his time at many Aboriginal community-controlled organisations, boards and committees. He was President of Indigenous Allied Health Australia in 2009–2010, Chairperson of the Indigenous Allied Health Australia Network in 2008, Vice President of Indigenous Allied Health Australia in 2011 and a representative on the national 'Close the Gap' committee in 2008–2009. James has received many awards over the years, including the Alumni Accolade Award from the University of South Australia in 2018, and the national NAIDOC Scholar of the Year in 2017 for his teaching, research and work in the Aboriginal community. He received the 2017 Faculty of Science, PVC Student Learning Student Experience Survey Award for his teaching in podiatry at Charles Sturt University. In 2014, James received the Golden Microscope Award from the Rotary Indigenous Health Foundation for his innovative foot and ankle work and his research in Aboriginal foot health.

MICHAEL CURTIN

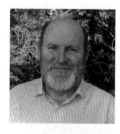

Michael Curtin is currently the Head of the School of Community Health at Charles Sturt University. He is an occupational therapist by background and has worked in this role in a number of different countries and communities. He is passionate about the rights of people to actively participate in activities and occupations that are personally meaningful. He believes that allied health professionals have to focus on the sociocultural and political contexts of their practice, as these contexts significantly impact on opportunities for people to engage in meaningful activities and occupations.

SALLY DRUMMOND

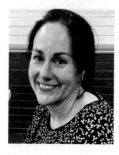

Sally Drummond is a Credentialed Mental Health Nurse with more than 20 years' experience in mental health and counselling, having held senior positions within the public and private healthcare and human services sectors. Sally currently works for

Charles Sturt University and CareSouth. Sally is also a highly experienced educationalist in the tertiary sector, with a focus on mental health, nursing and Indigenous health. Sally has interests in working with clients across the lifespan and their families regarding a wide range of mental health concerns, as well as mental health nursing, trauma-informed practice development, workplace learning, service delivery, and rural and remote health. She has a particular passion for clinical supervision, infant, child and adolescent mental health, and Indigenous health and firmly believes that working with individuals, groups and communities empowers them to find their unique solutions and truly flourish, leading to sustainable outcomes that will give rise to intergenerational change.

NORMAN DULVARIE

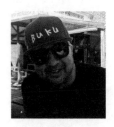

Norman Dulvarie (Milika Dhamarandji) came from Boigu Island, part of the top-western group of the Torres Strait Islands and the most northerly inhabited island of Australia. He said that 'I also have cultural ties to North East Arnhem Land. I have family everywhere.' He became an Aboriginal Health Worker in 1995 and a registered nurse in 2010. He later worked as a registered Aboriginal Health Practitioner for the Albury Wodonga Aboriginal Health Service and the Remote Area Health Corps. He said that he loved his job because 'I really love helping people. In my spare time I enjoy being with my two children, plus cycling, fishing, camping and Netflix.'

SIMONE GRAY

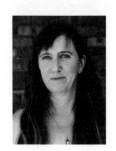

Simone Gray has been working with the School of Indigenous Australian Studies at Charles Sturt University for more than seven years. She has a Bachelor of Arts (English and Sociology) from the Australian National University. Simone gained employment in Aboriginal Education and Aboriginal Employment Policy Units within the Australian Public Service. After taking time off to raise a family, she worked in various roles including Indigenous student engagement and retention at a Dubbo primary school for seven years. Simone recently completed a Master of Arts (Journalism) with a focus specifically on Aboriginal issues. Simone's cultural knowledge has been gained through experience, including learning from her extended Aboriginal and Tongan family. Simone hopes for greater understanding of Australia's shared history and that knowledge, understanding and an appreciation of Aboriginal and Torres Strait Islander peoples' cultures will allow for meaningful reconciliation in this country.

AMALI HOHOL

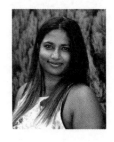

Amali Hohol is a Lecturer in Nursing in the School of Nursing, Midwifery and Indigenous Health at Charles Sturt University and has extensive experience teaching in the undergraduate nursing program. She has more than 13 years of industry experience specialising in intensive care and cardiovascular nursing.

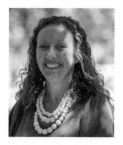

FAYE MCMILLAN

Associate Professor Faye McMillan is a Wiradjuri yinaa (woman) from Trangie in NSW. Faye is a Senior Atlantic Fellow for Social Equity (inaugural cohort) and was a founding member of Indigenous Allied Health Australia (IAHA). Faye works at Charles Sturt University as the Director of the Djirruwang Program—Bachelor of Health Science (Mental Health). Faye holds a Doctor of Health Science, a Master of Indigenous Health Studies and Bachelor of Pharmacy, and is Australia's first registered Aboriginal pharmacist. She also holds Graduate Certificates in Indigenous Governance from the University of Arizona (USA) and Wiradjuri Language, Culture and Heritage (CSU), and a Graduate Certificate in Education from the University of Melbourne's Graduate School of Education. In 2018 and 2019 Faye was a finalist in the NSW Women of the Year Awards, in 2017 she was recognised in the Who's Who of Australian Women, and in 2014 she was included in the Australian Financial Review and Westpac 100 Women of Influence.

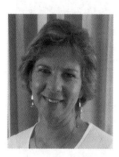

AMANDA MOSES

Amanda Moses holds a Bachelor of Nursing from Deakin University, a Graduate Diploma in Oncology Nursing from the Australian Catholic University and a Masters of Nursing (Nurse Practitioner) from the University of Newcastle.

She has more than 30 years' nursing experience in a range of metropolitan, rural and remote locations and settings, including intensive care, coronary care, paediatrics, community health, surgical care and acute medical care. An interest in primary and community health has led to a specific focus on rural and remote areas, including oncology nursing. A passion for improving the quality of life for persons with chronic and complex conditions resulted in Amanda following the path to become an endorsed Nurse Practitioner, with a scope of practice in chronic disease management. Amanda now lectures at Charles Sturt University, teaching undergraduate Primary Health Care and Chronic Disease Management, and postgraduate Chronic Disease Management and Clinical Education subjects.

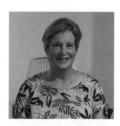

AILSA MUNNS

Ailsa Munns is a Registered Nurse, Registered Midwife and Child Health Nurse who has been working in community health for 40 years in urban, rural and remote areas. She is currently teaching child and adolescent health nursing at Curtin University. Her research interests include child and adolescent nursing practice, parent support for Aboriginal and non-Indigenous families, and the prevention of childhood anaemia in rural and remote Aboriginal communities.

OXFORD UNIVERSITY PRESS

MARYANNE PODHAM

Maryanne Podham is a Lecturer in Nursing at Charles Sturt University, and has a passion for student-centred education and continuous improvement in clinical practices. She has more than 25 years' experience in clinical, education and management nursing roles in rural NSW.

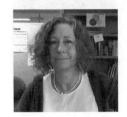

CAROLINE ROBINSON

Caroline Robinson is the Associate Professor Podiatry and Associate Head of School of Community Health at Charles Sturt University. Previously she has worked as a course director and developed experience in quality assurance for curriculum, learning and teaching across a range of undergraduate and postgraduate health courses. Caroline's collaboration with the School of Indigenous Australian Studies and the Gulaay Indigenous Australian Curriculum and Resources Team at CSU informs her work in scaffolding Indigenous Australian content in courses to facilitate students' Indigenous cultural competence journey. As a non-Indigenous academic, Caroline's cultural competence journey has been enabled by collaboration with Aboriginal and non-Aboriginal colleagues; participation in an on-country immersion at Menindee Lakes, NSW; completion of the 'Aboriginal Sydney' MOOC at the University of Sydney; participation in the LIME VII conference in 2017; and completion of the CSU Indigenous Cultural Competence training program. Her interests include whole-of-course assessment in relation to the Indigenous curriculum and also the concept of 'care' in health curricula. Caroline's current research is related to academic staff cultural competence in relation to learning and teaching and developing cultural competence for allied health students.

KRISTY ROBSON

Kristy Robson is a podiatry academic and researcher in the School of Community Health at Charles Sturt University. She has been working as a podiatrist and academic in regional and rural Australia her entire professional career. Kristy lectures in paediatrics within the podiatry program at CSU and is also the co-coordinator of an interprofessional paediatric disability placement in Vietnam for final year allied health students. This placement program was nationally recognised with an Australia Office of Learning and Teaching Award in 2014. Kristy is regularly invited to be a visiting scholar at international institutions presenting on a range of paediatric-related conditions.

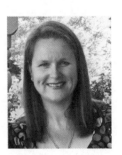

MEGAN SMITH

Megan Smith is the Executive Dean of the Faculty of Science at Charles Sturt University. Megan joined CSU in 1999 as an inaugural member of the team that developed the first rurally based physiotherapy program in Australia. Originally from the Riverina in NSW, she practised as a clinical physiotherapist in metropolitan Australia and the UK before returning to the bush to pursue an academic career. During her time at CSU she has held numerous leadership roles including Head of the School of Community

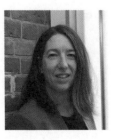

Health. Megan contributed strongly to the successful bid to establish a University Department of Rural Health at CSU and is the inaugural Director of the Three Rivers UDRH. Megan's research and teaching interests are in delivering high-quality health professional education. Her goal is to positively impact on the lives of people whose preference, like hers, is to live, work and study in rural Australia.

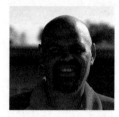

DARREN WIGHTON

Darren Wighton is a 49-year-old Wiradjuri man from Condobolin, a community leader and an artist. He is married to Michelle with two teenage sons and has worked in pastoral care and Aboriginal health. He is currently in Catholic Education.

OXFORD UNIVERSITY PRESS

INTRODUCTION

Aboriginal and Torres Strait Islander peoples' health has been written about, discussed and theorised on for many years. Primarily this has been in response to poorer health outcomes that have been attributed to a range of factors. Approaches to healthcare by Aboriginal and Torres Strait Islander peoples have been in place for over 40,000 years. Recognised as one of the oldest cultures in the world, healthcare practices are sustainable, holistic and effective. However, mainstream healthcare within Australia has not always been responsive to these ways. A move to reorient mainstream health to Aboriginal and Torres Strait Islander peoples' ways is paramount and timely. Research has clearly demonstrated that mainstream approaches to Aboriginal and Torres Strait Islander peoples' health are largely ineffectual and have unearthed intrinsic bias, stereotypes and racism (Larson, Coffin, Gilles & Howard, 2007).

Key leaders in Aboriginal and Torres Strait Islander people's health are making positive steps in ensuring the opportunities for health and wellness within communities are optimal. In 2018, we saw the implementation of cultural safety into the Australian nursing and midwifery standards (2018). This is a commitment to closing the health disparity gap by 2031 (Close the Gap Campaign Steering Committee, 2018) and importantly prioritises skills development, attitudes and behaviours of Australian health professionals as a way forward. Within the universities sector, Universities Australia implemented the Indigenous Cultural Competency Framework in collaboration with the Indigenous Higher Education Advisory Council in 2014 to support best practice. As you will read in Chapters 1 and 3, disciplines are also striving to move forward in this important space.

As we will explore in Chapter 1, the skills behaviours and attitudes of clinicians does impact healthcare outcomes, prioritising rapid development in health professionals' skills. Importantly, the lifelong journey of Indigenous Australian cultural competence can gear the non-Indigenous clinician to skills that will strengthen healthcare delivery and ensure that all Australians have equal and equitable access to healthcare.

Within Australia, we see trends in health and wellness for Aboriginal and Torres Strait Islander peoples being significantly below those of non-Indigenous people. For example, average life expectancy was estimated by the Commonwealth of Australia (2017) as being 9.5 years lower for Aboriginal and Torres Strait Islander females and 10.6 years lower for Aboriginal and Torres Strait Islander males. Alarmingly, key areas of health outcomes are similar to those of developing countries (Close the Gap Campaign Steering Committee, 2018). However, within communities we see strength, resilience and wisdom.

Importantly, we believe that our focus must not always be oriented to the deficit but instead to the strengths we find in communities. Aboriginal and Torres Strait Islander peoples' cultures have been built on the foundations of strength and resilience for families and communities through the strong connection to country. As discussed in Chapter 3, Aboriginal and Torres Strait Islander peoples' concepts of health and wellbeing are based on a holistic approach to healthcare that includes the connection to family, kin and community, and to country, culture, spirituality and ancestry. It is fundamental that the wider health system learns, understands and embraces the importance of holistic social and emotional wellbeing.

This textbook has been written using a strengths-based approach, with Indigenous Australian cultural competence and a reconciliation framework to health at the forefront. Each of these terms will be discussed at length within chapters. Each chapter has involved the collaboration of an Aboriginal or Torres Strait Islander and a non-Indigenous author representing the disciplines of nursing, midwifery and allied health. It was important for us to ensure that, as a writing team, we were on a pathway of Indigenous Australian cultural competence. We have learnt from and with each other over a period of 18 months. We encourage you to learn from your colleagues as you move into your profession. From the collective wisdom of each author, it is evident that when we are truly listening we can bring about change.

Deep listening often requires us to acknowledge difference. This brought us to the realisation that a reconciliation framework is critical. Reconciliation is a term that means something different to each individual. As defined by the Oxford English Dictionary (2017), it is the act of bringing together. Many groups within Australia have a unique and individual focus on reconciliation in regard to all Australian people, and by acknowledging and working through these different approaches we can make a significant and enduring difference to the health and wellbeing of Aboriginal and Torres Strait Islander peoples.

A WORD ON TERMINOLOGY

During European colonisation, using traditional Aboriginal and Torres Strait Islander languages was forbidden; instead, the language used was often discriminatory and inappropriate (NSW Department of Health, 2004). This is important to recognise, along with the evolving nature of language in Aboriginal and Torres Strait Islander peoples' cultures today. Terminology used in this text has been guided by the NSW Department of Health Communicating Positively guide (NSW Department of Health, 2004). The term 'Aboriginal and Torres Strait Islander peoples' reflects the diversity and plurality of the range of cultures alive in Australia today. By contrast, the term 'Indigenous Australian cultural competence' refers to the notion of clinicians considering how their values, beliefs and behaviour influence the care they provide to Aboriginal and Torres Strait Islander peoples. Given that there are over 270 nations within Australia, this term should be relevant to the practice of all clinicians, inclusive of practitioners who identify as Aboriginal or Torres Strait Islander.

REFERENCES

Australian Nursing and Midwifery Accreditation Council. (2018). *National guidelines for the accreditation of nursing and midwifery programs leading to registration and endorsement in Australia*. Canberra: ANMAC.

Close the Gap Campaign Steering Committee for Indigenous Health Equality. (2018). *A ten-year review: the Closing the Gap Strategy and Recommendations for Reset*. Retrieved from https://www.humanrights.gov.au/sites/default/files/document/publication/CTG%202018_FINAL-WEB.pdf

OXFORD UNIVERSITY PRESS

Commonwealth of Australia. (2017). *National strategic framework for Aboriginal and Torres Strait Islander peoples' mental health and social and emotional wellbeing.* Canberra: Department of the Prime Minister and Cabinet.

Larson, A., Coffin, J., Gilles, M., & Howard, P. (2007). It's enough to make you sick: The impact of racism on the health of Aboriginal Australians. *Australian and New Zealand Journal of Public Health, 34*(1), 322–328.

New South Wales Health. (2004). *Communicatively positively guide.* Retrieved from https://www.health.nsw.gov.au/aboriginal/publications/pub-terminology.pdf

Reconciliation. (2017). In A. Stevenson (Ed.). *Oxford dictionary of English* (3rd ed.). Oxford: Oxford University Press.

HOW TO USE THIS TEXTBOOK

Fostering inter-professional learning case studies, each chapter will provide valuable insight into health professionals' skills in specific areas. Part 1 of the text will introduce theoretical concepts that will support your learning and development. Part 2 of the text will raise your awareness and understanding in specific health domains. As previously discussed, the textbook is co-authored by an Aboriginal or Torres Strait Islander Australian author working alongside non-Indigenous authors, modelling a reconciliation framework. Case studies explore the real-life stories of Aboriginal and Torres Strait Islander community members, and we encourage readers to take the time to meaningfully engage with the journey of the individual in each case study.

This textbook has been endorsed by local community Elders following Aboriginal and Torres Strait Islander peoples' protocols prior to publication. This text highlights strengths and concerns in communities, providing an opportunity for learners to progress their thinking and approach to care. The text has been approved by Aboriginal and Torres Strait Islander community working parties as being culturally appropriate to disseminate. Also, we acknowledge that Aboriginal and Torres Strait Islander peoples are not a homogenous group and the perspectives on health and wellbeing discussed in this textbook do not speak on behalf of all Aboriginal and Torres Strait Islander communities.

Most importantly, this textbook is one learning opportunity. We encourage your journey of Indigenous Australian cultural competence to be broad, lifelong and varied. This textbook will not address all of your questions. It will, however, prove to be a unique learning opportunity for you to connect with Aboriginal and Torres Strait Islander peoples' health in an authentic and meaningful way. We encourage you to walk forward with compassion, seeking the truth and ensuring that your clients' voices are heard.

ACKNOWLEDGMENTS

There are many people to thank in the writing of this textbook. Importantly, we thank all contributors for their time, knowledge and expertise. This text would not have been possible without your wisdom and commitment. To community members that have shared their stories with bravery and honesty, we thank you.

We would like to thank our two children, Stella and Audrey, for their support, interest and understanding while we attended to this text. You keep us grounded and help us navigate the important aspects of our world.

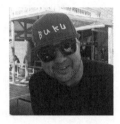

During the writing of this textbook, a friend, colleague and author passed away suddenly. Norman Dulvarie had a passion for nursing that supported the strength in Aboriginal and Torres Strait Islander communities. Norman was from Boigu Island in the Torres Strait Islands and had cultural ties to North East Arnhem Land. He walked with communities, sharing a pathway to stronger health outcomes.

We celebrate that his passion and skills have been shared in this textbook.

OXFORD UNIVERSITY PRESS

GUIDED TOUR

Each chapter begins with **learning concepts** to help you focus on the chapter's core knowledge, attitudes and skills to be learnt within the chapter. These concepts are linked and expanded upon in each end-of-chapter **summary** to consolidate your learning.

LEARNING CONCEPTS

Studying this chapter should enable you to:

1. identify the national prevalence of endocrine disorders in Aboriginal and Torres Strait Islander communities.
2. identify the risk factors of endocrine disorders in Aboriginal and Torres Strait Islander communities.
3. discuss the role nurses and allied healthcare team members can play to provide management options, promote healthy behaviours and effectively communicate with Aboriginal and Torres Strait Islander people with an endocrine disorder using safe and culturally appropriate strategies.

SUMMARY

This chapter has introduced the complexities associated with Aboriginal and Torres Strait Islander peoples' endocrinological health and wellness. When considering the burden of endocrine diseases in Aboriginal and Torres Strait Islander peoples through the key learning concepts, the role of health promotion and education is vital for nurses and allied health professionals.

Learning concept 1

Identify the national prevalence of endocrine disorders in Aboriginal and Torres Strait Islander communities: There is a high prevalence of endocrine disorders in Aboriginal and Torres Strait Islander communities, particularly type 2 diabetes, which is reported to be the second leading cause of death among Aboriginal and Torres Strait Islander peoples.

KEY TERMS

allied health professionals

empowerment

endocrine disorder

health literacy

metabolic syndrome

Key terms help you pinpoint important concepts that you need to know to be an effective and competent healthcare professional. These terms are listed at the beginning of each chapter, defined in **margin notes** where they first appear, and collated in the **glossary** at the end of the book.

health literacy Personal skills, knowledge, motivation and capacity to access, understand and use information to make decisions about one's own health and healthcare choices.

Health literacy needs to be viewed within two separate aspects: the health literacy of an individual, and the environment in which health literacy is being delivered. For an individual to improve their health literacy there needs to be a clear interplay between these two elements. The Australian Commission on Safety and Quality in Health Care suggests that health literacy involves a person's abilities and skills to find, analyse and adopt information to address their health needs. Further, the ability of the person to

GLOSSARY

Aboriginal Community Controlled Health Service (ACCHS)
A primary healthcare service initiated and operated by a local Aboriginal community to deliver holistic, comprehensive and culturally appropriate healthcare to the community, which controls it through a locally elected board made up of Aboriginal people.

critical reflection
A deep form of reflective learning that creates the opportunity for our worldviews to be transformed.

culture
A set of common beliefs, attitudes and norms shared by a group.

IMPLICATIONS FOR NURSING AND ALLIED HEALTH PRACTICE

The Registered Nurse Code of Conduct and the Professional Standards have defined professional conduct and behaviours to ensure that all consumers of healthcare are able to access care. Review these standards.

Similarly, every registered allied health professional must follow their respective code of conduct. Within in each code of conduct, behaviour regarding race, racism and discrimination is mandated. Review your professional code of conduct.

Implications for practice boxes provide practical examples or explanations to show how health and societal factors impact on healthcare practice.

Case studies throughout the chapters provide person-centred scenarios similar to those you will come across in your career as a healthcare professional. These studies and the accompanying **critical reflection questions** allow you to reflect on your learning and practice, putting your knowledge to use in a realistic healthcare scenario.

Case study 2.1: General healthcare

Denise's story

Denise is a woman of Anglo heritage who admits herself to the birthing room at her local hospital. She gives birth to a son with blonde hair and blue eyes. Her partner attends the birth and they proceed to discuss the two options to name their son—Connor or Djarra. The midwife and doctor exchange puzzled looks, so the mother explains that her partner is of Aboriginal heritage and therefore so is their son. They decide on the name Djarra and then have to explain its origins from a family language dictionary. A day later, after receiving the paperwork to be released to go home, Denise realises that the form has changed. She had ticked the box stating that her son was to identify as Aboriginal, but the tick has been removed. She queries the nursing staff, whose response is that they thought she had made a mistake. Denise is embarrassed and angry.

CRITICAL REFLECTION QUESTIONS

- Why do you think Denise felt this way?
- What message does this send to the family from the nursing staff?
- Thinking about the power relations, how do you think you would have approached the identity of the child?

Revision questions will help you think deeply about issues covered in each chapter, to prepare you for assessment and practice.

REVISION QUESTIONS

1. Explain how this chapter links to the Australian Registered Nurse Code of Professional Conduct and Code of Ethics in Nursing.
2. In your own words explain what the evidence-based research indicates are the physiological impacts of negative behaviours that are directed towards a person's race.

REFERENCES

Ahn, J. W. (2017). Structural equation modeling of cultural competence of nurses caring for foreign patients. *Asian Nursing Research*, 11(1), 65-73.

Almutairi, A. F., Adlan, A. A., & Nasim, M. (2017). Perceptions of the critical cultural competence of registered nurses in Canada. *BMC Nursing*, 16(1), 47.

FURTHER READINGS/ADDITIONAL RESOURCES

Albury Wodonga Aboriginal Health Service: https://www.awahs.com.au
National Aboriginal Community Controlled Health Organisation: https://www.naccho.org.au
Orange Aboriginal Medical Service: https://www.oams.net.au

Along with the **references**, **further readings/additional resources** are provided to help you identify further resources to support your learning.

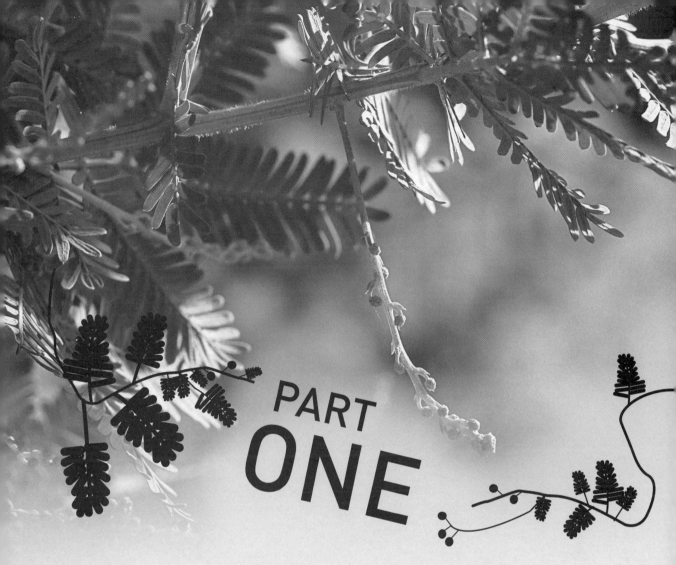

PART
ONE

Frameworks for health and competence

This section will introduce key theoretical and historical concepts that will enable your development and growth in Aboriginal and Torres Strait Islander peoples' healthcare. This section is important to consider prior to embarking on health systems knowledge.

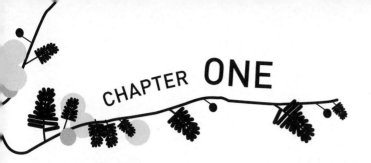

CHAPTER **ONE**

Indigenous Australian cultural competence

Jessica Biles and Brett Biles

LEARNING CONCEPTS

Studying this chapter should enable you to:

1. identify the importance of Indigenous Australian cultural competence.
2. identify the historical context behind Indigenous Australian cultural competence.
3. identify the importance of skills that enable the journey of Indigenous Australian cultural competence.
4. determine strategies that promote Indigenous Australian cultural competence in practice.
5. identify your own professional plan in Indigenous Australian cultural competence.

KEY TERMS

critical reflection
culture
Indigenous Australian cultural competence
transcultural care
worldview

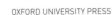

Introduction

Indigenous Australian cultural competence
A nonlinear process in which non-Indigenous health workers consider how their values, beliefs and behaviour influence the care they provide to Aboriginal and Torres Strait Islander peoples.

This chapter will encourage you to begin thinking about the relevance of **Indigenous Australian cultural competence**.

Throughout this chapter you will be asked to reflect on and consider what culture and cultural competence means to you as a registered nurse and/or allied health practitioner. This will involve considering what defines culture, the history and significance of Indigenous Australian cultural competence, and finally how cultural competence translates into clinical practice. Often the lifelong journey of cultural competence can be challenging. It requires us to reflect on our beliefs, attitudes and values—on the very essence of who we are as a person—and then consider how these may influence, change or enhance the care we provide to our clients. This can be an uncomfortable process. Often in times of discomfort we learn and are more inclined to retain the learning.

critical reflection
A deep form of reflective learning that creates the opportunity for our worldviews to be transformed.

This chapter will require you to reflect. Reflecting critically on yourself as a person in a diverse world and as a clinician is vital to enacting Indigenous Australian cultural competence. Case studies will be provided to encourage **critical reflection**, and links to other sections of this textbook will help to provide professional context.

The importance of Indigenous Australian cultural competence within the Australian health landscape

Historically health outcomes for Aboriginal and Torres Strait Islander peoples have been significantly worse than for non-Indigenous Australian people (Australian Bureau of Statistics, 2012, 2015). This has been addressed by many different government and non-government initiatives. The most prominent campaign was introduced in 2008 when the Australian government recognised the need to make the changes required to reduce health disparities by funding the development of the Close the Gap campaign. This campaign was, and remains, important for a variety of reasons. It showed the wider health community the gravity of health disparities in all areas of Aboriginal and Torres Strait Islander peoples' health and healthcare (Council of Australian Governments (COAG) Reform Council, 2010) and enabled an opportunity to report successes as initiatives were implemented.

The Closing the Gap campaign was supported by the *National Strategic Framework for Aboriginal and Torres Strait Islander Health 2003–2013*, which had an overarching philosophy of ensuring equality in cultural considerations in care, and of dignity and justice underpinning health. This framework was later progressed to the *National*

Aboriginal and Torres Strait Islander Health Plan 2013–2023 (Commonwealth of Australia, 2013). This plan importantly focused on not only health priorities but also principles in healthcare delivery, and highlighted a vision for the eradication of systemic and non-systemic racism in healthcare within Australia.

Racism will be further explored in Chapter 2, but it is important to create links in this foundational chapter in relation to Indigenous Australian cultural competence. In this era we are in a position to look back and see some positive changes in Aboriginal and Torres Strait Islander peoples' morbidity and mortality. In data collated from 1998 to 2013 by the Australian Bureau of Statistics, we can see a decrease in mortality. Although this can be viewed as a positive shift, there is still much work to be done as a nation (see differences in mortality rates between Indigenous and non-Indigenous populations in Figure 1.1). The exploration of morbidity and mortality brings our attention to healthcare and healthcare outcomes. It also raises the notions of health professionals' attitudes, biases and understandings of Aboriginal and Torres Strait Islander peoples' concepts of health and connections to Australian health providers. A United Nations thematic paper highlighted the need to provide equality in healthcare for Aboriginal and Torres Strait Islander peoples (Inter-Agency Support Group on Indigenous Peoples' Issues, 2014).

Several thoughts have been raised as to why the health gap still exists, particularly with current government strategy, funding allocations and raised awareness of health disparity (Australian Institute of Health and Welfare, 2016). Various rationales have been revealed over the course of many years of research in this important area. While

Figure 1.1 Age distribution of deaths, by age, sex and Indigenous status, NSW, Qld, WA, SA and NT combined, 2008–2012

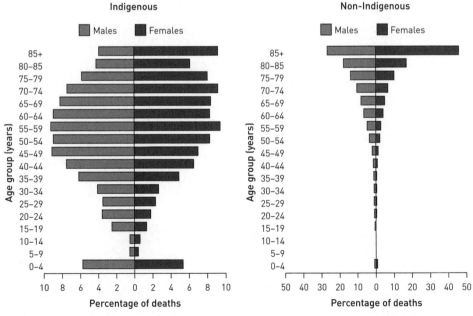

Source: Australian Institute of Health and Welfare (2014).

we continue to learn in this area, we do have some insight that health outcomes of Aboriginal and Torres Strait Islander peoples have been linked to four important areas:

- socio-economic disadvantage
- a lack of culturally appropriate healthcare resources used in mainstream health
- Western models of healthcare being the primary model of care provided within mainstream healthcare in Australia
- a lack of confidence in accessing healthcare early in a period of illness or at all due to direct and indirect racism by healthcare providers (Larson, Gillies, Howard & Coffin, 2007; Kidd, Watts & Saltman, 2008; Maher, 2013).

Therefore, our actions, thoughts and beliefs as health professionals are important in the delivery of healthcare and can result in a change in healthcare outcomes for our clients. This forms foundational thinking about the importance of Indigenous Australian cultural competence within Australia.

Studies (Durey, Thompson & Wood, 2011; Taylor, Thompson & Davis, 2010) have revealed that Aboriginal and Torres Strait Islander peoples are more likely to access healthcare when communication is respectful, where clinicians have an understanding of Aboriginal and Torres Strait Islander peoples' cultures, and where clinicians are able to work towards the development of good relationships that involve Aboriginal and Torres Strait Islander health workers as a part of the healthcare team. It is important that health professionals have the skills, attitudes and beliefs to ensure this is achievable within Australian healthcare facilities.

It has been cited by many that mandatory training in the area of Aboriginal and Torres Strait Islander peoples' health may result in better health outcomes for consumers of healthcare (Health Workforce Australia, 2011). In 2016, the release of the *Aboriginal and Torres Strait Islander Health Curriculum Framework* (Commonwealth of Australia, 2016) provided evidence and support for health practitioners embedding content into undergraduate courses (discussed further in Chapter 3). The implementation of Aboriginal and Torres Strait Islander content into courses is thought to provide much-needed training and development in the area of Indigenous Australian cultural competence. Most importantly, we must highlight that short courses have proved to have little effect on sustainable personal changes that may influence the care we provide to clients (Paul, Carr & Milroy, 2006). Therefore, models of learning need to be considered across a lengthy period of time, perhaps even a lifetime.

Case study 1.1: Nursing focus

John's story

John is a nurse employed at a major health service. He has recently been to a professional development course that focused on Indigenous Australian cultural competence. The training consisted of an online module and a face-to-face workshop with colleagues he knows well. As he was leaving the training, a registered nurse colleague came up to him and said, 'This training is so pointless—what a waste of time! I don't care how people think or behave. As long as they get the medical treatment I am happy. The rest is just politeness, which I do not have time for. They always end up coming back anyway.' John was surprised at his colleague's attitude to care and the training program. He decided to grab himself a coffee before heading back to the ward. He wanted to reflect on the situation he had just encountered and consider its meaning in nursing practice.

CRITICAL REFLECTION QUESTIONS

- What are your initial responses to this situation?
- What are the benefits and risks raised for John (personally), to the healthcare service and to the public?
- How might John proceed in this situation? What key practice considerations arise?
- What might be other considerations when viewing this case study?

Case study 1.2: Allied health focus

Jacinta's story

Jacinta is the manager of the Allied Health Department at a major public health service. Jacinta has been tasked with reviewing the statistics of Aboriginal and Torres Strait Islander people accessing the Allied Health Department over the last two years and with providing a presentation to her manager. Jacinta decided to approach the team leaders of each allied health discipline to seek their support in putting together the statistics.

Jacinta spoke with Rob the physiotherapy team leader who said, 'This will be an easy report for the physio team as hardly any Aboriginal and Torres Strait Islander people access the physiotherapy services.' Jacinta did not reply to Rob's comments, but as she was walking to her office she started reflecting on them. Jacinta then spoke with Sarah, the occupational therapy team leader, and Sarah's comments were very similar to Rob's. Jacinta was concerned that both team leaders made very similar comments and was unsure how to proceed.

(Continued)

Jacinta decided to have a yarn with Jason, the Aboriginal community liaison officer, about both Rob's and Sarah's comments. Jason responded to Jacinta by simply saying, 'How do Rob and Sarah know if Indigenous people access the allied health services?'

Jacinta thanked Jason for his time and advice, and decided to go away and reflect on his comments before speaking with Rob and Sarah again.

CRITICAL REFLECTION QUESTIONS

- What are your initial responses to this situation?
- How might Jacinta proceed in this situation? What key practice considerations arise?
- What might be other considerations when viewing this case study?

The history of Indigenous Australian cultural competence

To understand cultural competence it is important that we consider where cultural competence was first developed and why. The term first emerged in the 1980s in the USA. It was particularly prevalent with teachers, social workers, and health and welfare workers as they were seeking ways to better meet the needs of multicultural communities. Although the term has been used within literature for some time, the implementation of cultural competency skills has been varied.

In the context of health, there was significant evidence that revealed people from ethnic and racial minorities experienced significantly poorer health outcomes than people from the majority/dominant culture (Betancourt, 2003; Brach & Fraser, 2000). While a range of biomedical models have explored why this may have occurred, it has taken time to shift our thinking from the 'problem patient' to what we can do, say, be or change to adapt our practice to each individual client and respond to their cultural, spiritual, social and physical needs. The concept of 'cultural competence' has since been a focus in Western English-speaking countries with Indigenous populations. A vast amount of literature about cultural competence has been generated mainly from the USA and Canada (Truong, Paradies & Priest, 2014; Clifford, McCalman, Bainbridge & Tsey, 2015), with an increasing body of work from Australia.

The literature indicates that while the term is used frequently, there remains confusion over the definition. Within healthcare a consensus has not been reached over the definition of 'cultural competence'. However, many definitions share key elements (Betancourt, Green & Carillo, 2002). These elements include but are not limited to the following: valuing diversity; having the capacity for cultural self-assessment; being conscious of the dynamics inherent in cross-cultural interactions; institutionalising the importance of cultural knowledge; and making adaptations to service delivery that reflect cultural understanding (Humphery, 2000; Ranzijn, McConnochie, Day, Nolan & Wharton, 2008). In other words, there are many models that suggest ways that nursing and allied health practitioners can become more culturally competent.

The language of cultural competence has created discussion. The very nature of the language assumes that the journey and learning have an end point (competence), and requires certain parameters to be obeyed. However, more recent models within Australia have indicated that cultural competence does not have an end point, and nor is it linear—instead, it is reliant on skill attributes and transformative learning. It has been shown that the journey is complex, occurs across a career and stimulates a change in an individual's viewpoint (Biles, Coyle, Bernoth & Hill, 2016). There are many ways that one can learn cultural competence skills and the learning can occur in many different ways. What seems to be common across the literature is that the cultural competence needs to be viewed as a journey that may never reach an end point (Hains, Lynch & Winton, 2000).

Models of cultural competence

As suggested earlier in this chapter, there are many ways that one can learn cultural competence. Models have been developed over time to assist in the delivery of cultural competence within undergraduate degrees. These models can focus on individual approaches as well as institutional approaches to the journey of cultural competence (Cross, Bazron, Dennis & Isaacs, 1989; Campinha-Bacote, 2002) to bring much-needed training in the area of cultural diversity. It would be useful to explore your own university's take on cultural competence.

Other Western nations such as America and Canada have a specific perspective on cultural competence. There seems to be a focus on both institutional and individual competence. These models emphasise that the development of cultural competence involves a two-way learning process. The process may be between the organisation and the individual or between the health professional and client (Campinha-Bacote, 2002). Cultural competence is much more than awareness; rather it is a philosophical approach to healthcare that influences the delivery of health services (National Health & Medical Research Council, 2005).

Wells (2000) writes from an American perspective and explains cultural competence via a continuum. The continuum is represented through a matrix that can guide the practitioner and their institution through a range of stages that are thought to promote competence. The matrix views the continuum as culturally incompetent to culturally proficient. Cultural proficient is detailed as being at the top of the matrix and does allude to an end point of competence. Many Australian universities embrace the Wells model of competence. Ranzijn et al. (2008) outline the important implications of the Wells model, explaining that the practice of cultural competence is about being sequential and fluid (able to move through stages at any time), highlighting that 'one-off' cultural awareness workshops are ineffectual.

Recent research in Australia has indicated that cultural competence training has resulted in an increased preparedness to work with Aboriginal people (Paul et al., 2006; McRae, Taylor, Swain & Sheldrake, 2008), a greater understanding of health challenges for Aboriginal and Torres Strait Islander peoples (Mooney, Bauman, Westwood, Kelaher, Tibben & Jalaludin, 2005) and improved relationships between Aboriginal and Torres Strait Islander peoples and non-Indigenous Australians, all of which can enhance access to services (Si, Bailie, Togni, Abbs & Robinson, 2006). Education of Australian health professionals in cultural competence is believed to be paramount (Hunt, Ramjan, McDonald, Koch, Baird & Salamonson, 2015).

Professions play a key role in the development and understanding of cultural competence (Ranzijn et al., 2008). For example, the Australian Nursing & Midwifery Accreditation Council (2015) has mandated the inclusion of a core subject in all undergraduate Bachelor of Nursing courses. It can be argued that the inclusion of a core subject requires educators to be on a journey of cultural competence. The onus is on educators providing learning opportunities to educate and prepare nurses for delivering their services in culturally appropriate ways, as well as preparing themselves to deliver education in a culturally responsive way. Achieving this requires support at an organisational level (Grote, 2008), something which many universities are still striving to achieve. Consider the opportunities that are presented to you as a current university student.

Professional organisations and Indigenous Australian cultural competence

Importantly, the Congress of Aboriginal and Torres Strait Islander Nurses and Midwives was established in 1997 with aims to address the health gap between Indigenous and non-Indigenous Australian people. The Congress has been responsible for many policies and recommendations guiding the development of nursing curriculum and best practice. The Congress released a statement in 2017 supporting the ongoing development of cultural safety of staff, students and healthcare services, recognising that this does rely on parity in the nursing and midwifery workforce (CATSINaM, 2017, pp. 11–12). It can be suggested that there is an interrelationship between cultural safety and cultural competence. To be cultural safe, practitioners need to be responsive to culture and on a journey of cultural competence.

Indigenous Allied Health Australia (IAHA) was established in 2009 from a network of allied health professionals, and in 2013 registered as a company. IAHA believes that Aboriginal and Torres Strait Islander health professionals play a major role in healthcare. In order to make a difference in health outcomes, the health workforce needs to be culturally responsive (IAHA, 2017).

> [IAHA] asserts that a culturally responsive health workforce is imperative in order to ensure Aboriginal and Torres Strait Islander people receive the healthcare required to significantly improve health and wellbeing outcomes. IAHA views culturally responsive care as a cyclical and ongoing process, requiring regular self-reflection and proactive responses to the person, family or community with whom the interaction is occurring.
>
> IAHA (2015, p. 1)

We can assume that if we have a body of health professionals each on a journey of Indigenous Australian cultural competence, we can move forward as a culturally responsive workforce.

The following Australian definition of cultural competence has been drawn from the *Ngapartji-Ngapartji Yerra* report of the Indigenous Higher Education Advisory Council (IHEAC, 2007), a council that provides advice to the Australian government on higher education, research and training (IHEAC, 2007). This is currently the most widely accepted definition used in Australia:

> Cultural competence is the awareness, knowledge, understanding and sensitivity to other cultures combined with a proficiency to interact appropriately with people from those cultures in a way that is congruent with the behaviour and expectations that members of a distinctive culture recognise as appropriate among themselves. Cultural competence includes having an awareness of one's own culture in order to understand its cultural limitations as well as being open to cultural differences, cultural integrity and the ability to use cultural resources. It can be viewed as a non-linear and dynamic process which integrates and interlinks individuals with the organisation and its systems.
>
> IHEAC (2007, pp. 5, 34–38, and amended in 2011, IHEAC meeting and endorsed by the IHEAC Chair and Deputy Chair)

Cultural competence and cultural safety

Within Australia, the terms 'cultural competence' and 'cultural safety' are at times used interchangeably. In New Zealand, the term 'cultural safety' is often used in preference to 'cultural competence'. Cultural safety, as defined by Eckermann, Dowd, Chong, Nixon, Gray and Johnson (2006, p. 213) is:

> An environment that is safe for people: where there is no assault, challenge or denial of their identity, of who they are and what they need. It is about shared respect, shared meaning, shared knowledge and experience, of learning, living and working together with dignity and truly listening.

The introduction of this term into nursing education stimulated a national review of cultural safety in New Zealand in the early 1990s (Ramsden, 1990) and resulted in the embedding and recognising of cultural safety as a foundation tool in nursing practice. The focus of this concept is primarily on the experience of the client, empowering the model to be considered from both an institutional and individual level involving specific skills. This has been well detailed by Eckermann et al. (2006).

Essentially, cultural safety can be defined by the experiences of the recipient of care rather than being a tool for a practitioner to embed (Eckermann et al., 2006). It is seen to require the skill of reflecting on one's own cultural identity and then the recognition of the impact one's culture has on practice.

The Australian Health Practitioner Regulation Agency (2018) has defined cultural safety in Australia as 'the individual and institutional knowledge, skills, attitudes and competencies needed to deliver optimal health care for Aboriginal and Torres Strait Islander peoples', while the Congress of Aboriginal and Torres Strait Islander Nurses and Midwives (2018) defines cultural safety as:

> a philosophy of practice that is about how a health professional does something, not [just] what they do ... It is about how people are treated in society, not about their diversity as such, so its focus is on systemic and structural issues and on the social determinants of health ... Cultural safety represents a key philosophical shift from providing care regardless of difference, to care that takes account of peoples' unique needs. It requires nurses and midwives to undertake an ongoing process of self-reflection and cultural self-awareness, and an acknowledgement of how a nurse's/midwife's personal culture impacts on care.

Within Australia, it is paramount that we are able to provide services of care that are culturally safe. Cultural safety should be deemed 'safe' by the client—not the institution. Within health services it is also paramount that we have well-equipped health professionals that acknowledge their own position in the world and are on a journey of individual cultural competence. This enables a workforce that is culturally responsive to the needs of Aboriginal and Torres Strait Islander peoples.

How to start the lifelong journey of Indigenous Australian cultural competence

In order to commence your journey in Indigenous Australian cultural competence, an understanding of five major terms is vital: non-linear learning, culture, worldview, discomfort and critical reflection. These five components will provide context in how you may decide to progress your learning journey. Importantly, this is not a recipe for cultural competence; however, these five major terms may assist your development in this space.

Non-linear learning

As discussed earlier, a range of models have attempted to explain and provide examples of how we 'do' cultural competence in healthcare (Biles et al., 2016; Campinha-

Bacote, 2002; Ranzijn et al., 2008). All of these models are evidenced as assisting the development of skills, values and behaviours. Importantly, what is apparent is that the journey seems to be non-linear. There are times when we will be faced with challenging circumstances that create a rapid shift in our thinking—circumstances that detract from prior learning—and we see a decline in our skills and/or a considered meaningful approach to learning Indigenous Australian cultural competence. This is important to note. The learning journey may not be a perfect linear progression and that is okay. We all have unique experiences and challenges that shape who we are as clinicians, and this is essential given the diverse population of Australian health. The important aspect to remember is that the journey must be across a lifetime. Culture shapes society and identity and is not static; therefore, our journey in Indigenous Australian cultural competence will always be moving and will not have an end point. Our journey is also shaped by the infrastructure in which healthcare is delivered (this will be further discussed in Chapter 3).

Figure 1.2 and Figure 1.3 present two models of learning Indigenous Australian cultural competence.

Figure 1.2 The Ranzijn, McConnochie, Day, Nolan and Wharton model of cultural competence

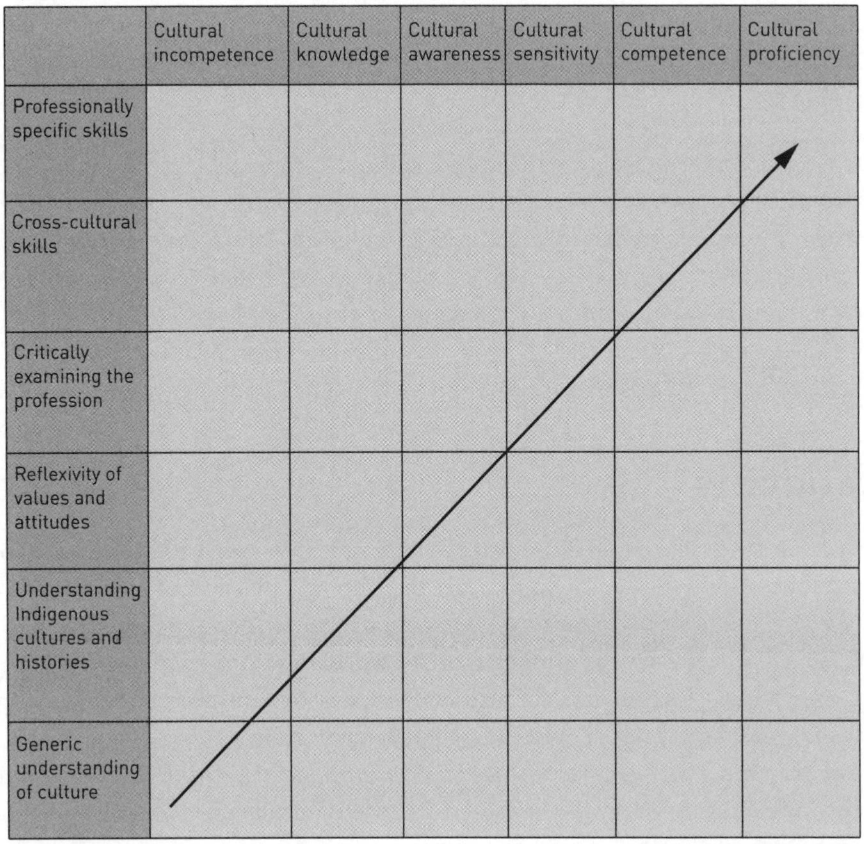

Source: Ranzijn et al. (2008).

Figure 1.3 The Biles, Coyle, Bernoth and Hill model of learning cultural competence in nursing

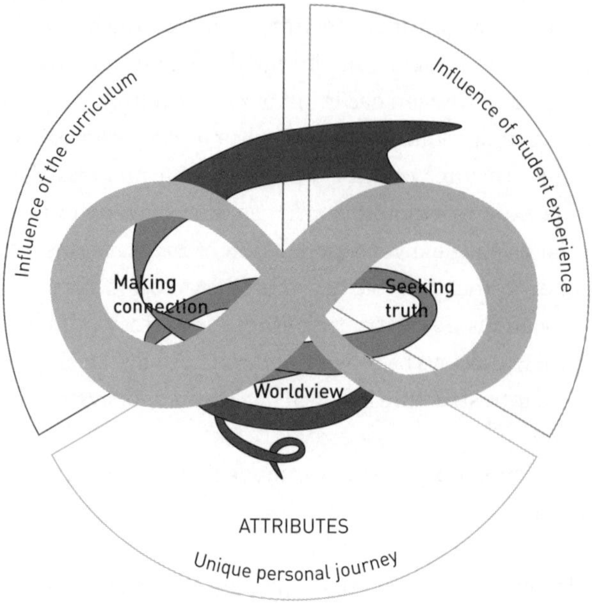

Influence of the curriculum

Influence of student experience

Making connection

Seeking truth

Worldview

ATTRIBUTES

Unique personal journey

Source: Biles (2017).

Culture

culture A set of common beliefs, attitudes and norms shared by a group.

When considering Indigenous Australian cultural competence, it is important to first consider our own **culture**. Culture has been defined as a set of common beliefs, attitudes and norms shared by a group (Ranzijn et al., 2008). Its definition moves culture beyond social rituals and traditions like artistic expressions and beliefs as being important to our worldview (discussed later in this chapter). Cultural groups shape their worldview and make the way that members live their lives 'right' for 'us' and different to others (Jenkins, 2006). Take a moment to consider your own culture.

Worldview

worldview How we see, are and react to the world around us.

Indigenous Australian cultural competence implores us to spend time navigating our own culture prior to being able to consider the cultural influences of another person. We are then in a position to reflect on our cultural position as a nurse or allied health professional. How we see the world shapes our **worldview**. Consider how you explore your own culture. Perhaps it is through discussion with your peers, reading a book, discussing your family ties or even through university study.

Worldview has been defined as a theoretical construct (Underhill, 2009), meaning that definitions of our worldview have been theorised and built upon over many decades shaping how we see, are and react to the world around us. There are many influences on our worldview that shape our norms, and often we are unaware that they exist until we experience difference. Difference may be around cultural norms, traditions, perspectives or gender, to name just a few (Best & Fredericks, 2014). Our worldview shapes how we see the world, how we engage with others and how we see difference (Payne & Payne, 2004). Our culture has the ability to influence our worldview.

Sociological perspectives around worldview suggest that the way in which we see ourselves in the world relates to cultural difference (Payne & Payne, 2004). An example of this is a specific dominant cultural group as discussed by Payne and Payne (2004), or other dominant groups such as male, heterosexual, white and middle class. Unconsciously, we often group together with others who share our sense of worldview and identity with the world. This can be challenging when considering difference and can promote the concept of 'othering' (Young, 2000). Othering is a challenging situation when we cluster towards our worldview groups and experience difference. We see the difference as 'other' and at times threatening to our sense of the world. It takes bravery to see the world in a different way and also it requires an element of discomfort.

Discomfort

There have been times when we have all felt discomfort. Perhaps the discomfort was during a dental appointment or a social situation where we were not comfortable with the group we were conversing with. Discomfort, which is not to be confused with distress, is an emotion where we feel unsettled, unnerved or slightly anxious (Merriam-Webster, 2017). Social theorist Megan Boler (2000) has discussed that this feeling of discomfort can promote an opportunity to feel and reconsider our own worldviews. The space where learning becomes uncomfortable can be a place where we reconsider the lens in which we see the world. Consider a workplace learning experience where you have felt discomfort. Did the experience enhance your learning and shift your thinking around a certain area?

When this occurs, it has the potential to enable us to reconsider and evaluate our own inner values. This space is important in Indigenous Australian cultural competence, where an Aboriginal or Torres Strait Islander person's view of health and wellness may differ from the personal view of a registered nurse or an allied health practitioner. Recognising these steps in your learning journey will assist not only in your practice but also in how you can relate to others in both your personal and professional world.

1. Consider a time that you have felt uncomfortable in both your personal and professional world. Record your memory of the feelings and the outcomes in your reflective journey.
2. List times that you have felt uncomfortable during clinical placement. Reflect on these situations and consider your learning during the situation.

Critical reflection

Critical reflection is a skill that is well recognised as being vital to both registered nurses and allied health practitioners (Jayatilleke & Mackie, 2013). Critical thinking has been defined as a metacognitive process requiring 'purposeful, insightful judgment that involves the development and effective utilisation of multiple dimensional cognitions to interpret and analyse a situation' (Facione & Facione, 2013, p. 6), arriving at an appropriate way to respond, act or reach a conclusion to a problem (Kaddoura, Van-Dyke & Yang, 2016). Both nursing and allied health practitioners have a range of models available to promote the use of critical thinking (Cottrell, 2017). Critical thinking has been shown to bring precision, accuracy and relevance to any given situation (Cottrell, 2017). It requires us to mindfully focus our attention on a situation, observe, identify key points, analyse and respond with the desired message (Cottrell, 2017).

Critical reflection is said to be a deep form of reflective learning that creates the opportunity for our worldviews to be transformed (Mezirow, 1981), linking with Indigenous Australian cultural competence. Mezirow (2010) describes transformative learning as the moment in time when you reconsider how you see the world, and also describes it as having the ability to challenge personal assumptions that may have an impact on professional worlds. For some learners it may be a particular learning experience such as clinical placement, and for others it may be a slower, more considered journey as they navigate their way through their undergraduate degree. Critical reflection is a vital competence in Indigenous Australian cultural competence. It creates the nexus to shift our thinking from our own norms and to start to think about the world through a different lens. Consider a learning experience that you have undertaken that has promoted a 'light bulb' moment. Perhaps the experience was through a conversation with a peer, a tutorial topic, a book or even a workplace learning situation. How did you feel and how did this influence your leaning?

Transcultural care—where does this fit?

Often when discussing Indigenous Australian cultural competence, the notion of **transcultural care** is raised. So, importantly, we must highlight where we see that it fits. This may assist your learning as an undergraduate student.

In the 1960s transcultural care was founded. Essentially transcultural care forms the knowledge, skills and behaviours that are responsive to the delivery of healthcare to more than one culture (Leininger, 1975; Leininger, 2002; Purnell & Paulanka, 2003). Leininger (2002) has written on the essence of nursing being 'care', and from this she links care to her model of transcultural nursing: the cultural care theory. This model has been used extensively in the development of nursing curricula (Leininger, 2002). Leininger (1975) suggests, and her model indicates, that the phenomenon of 'care' had

transcultural care
Knowledge, skills and behaviours that are responsive to the delivery of healthcare to more than one culture.

cultural contexts that were often not valued in the nursing profession. Leininger was foundational in nursing practice, raising attention on how culture influences the care we give and receive.

The purpose and goal of the cultural care theory is to provide culturally congruent, safe and meaningful care to clients of diverse or similar cultures (Leininger, 2002). The model is linear, cross-cultural and focuses on cognition, suggesting assessment techniques that are inclusive of 10 principles that practising clinicians should consider as a guide for practice (Leininger, 2002). Of interest, the model has been reinvigorated in teaching cultural competence in American nursing schools since the New York twin towers attack of 2001 (Leininger, 2002). One particularly important aspect in the cultural care theory is that it is believed that registered nurses and allied health professionals require an inner desire to practise transcultural nursing (Leininger, 1975). This is important and determines the success of the model's application.

Another model of transcultural nursing is the Purnell model of cultural competence. It originated in Canada and consists of 12 domains that are important for the nurse to consider, and relies on the nurse being able to assess using the domains within practice (Purnell & Paulanka, 2003). The Purnell model claims to have transcultural applications; however, the practice-based approach of the model reveals major assumptions that the underpinning of all cultures have similarities (Purnell & Paulanka, 2003), which does not always represent best care in all cultural contexts and is reliant on both organisations and individuals working together.

Transcultural care is important in Australian healthcare systems. There are similarities between the journey of Indigenous Australian cultural competence and the transcultural model of care. The skills in Indigenous Australian cultural competence are transferable to many cultural groups. The journey is driven from within the health professional.

IMPLICATIONS FOR NURSING AND ALLIED HEALTH PRACTICE

As registered nurses and allied health professionals we often experience situations with our clients when they are at their most vulnerable. It is important that our behaviours, skills and practices reflect diversity and respect the client's worldview rather than our own. Locate the Nursing and Midwifery Board's *Registered Nurse Standards for Practice* (2016) or your specific professional standards that relate to Indigenous Australian cultural competence. Review the standards and consider which standards you feel are appropriate to your learning journey.

Developing a professional plan will assist in your application and progression in Indigenous Australian cultural competence. As discussed earlier, the journey in Indigenous Australian cultural competence is across a lifetime. It may involve a range of activities that can be uncomfortable, and require critical reflection that promotes a sense of cultural identity in the world and an understanding of personal worldviews.

A professional plan evidences commitment, intention and thought into a specific area. It can align with professional standards or form a personal connection between ideas, thoughts and activities that are undertaken in a professional career. Consider what a professional portfolio may look like in your discipline area. Table 1.1 depicts one method of capturing professional goals in the area of Indigenous Australian cultural competence. A professional plan can be used in a professional portfolio, which is a requirement of all health practitioners in Australia and demonstrates that you are self-regulating your learning needs in a specific area.

Table 1.1 Professional plan for Indigenous Australian cultural competence

Professional standard	Personal activity	Professional activity	Reflective diary entry

Case study 1.3: Nursing focus

Sally's story

Sally is a student in an undergraduate nursing program in Australia. Sally has moved from a regional location to a metropolitan city to attend university. She lives on campus in shared accommodation and has made a large network of friends. Sally has been advised by her lecturers that her second placement is at a large metropolitan Aboriginal Health Service. She has recently completed a subject on Aboriginal and Torres Strait Islander peoples' health in her nursing degree program and obtained a credit in the subject. She enjoyed the learning, but struggled to grasp why it was required in a nursing degree. Now Sally needs to prepare herself for the placement. She has mixed emotions of excitement and apprehension. She shares some of her feelings with her friends, who do not understand her apprehension. Sally is confused by her feelings and has decided to complete some additional study on her own to prepare for her placement.

CRITICAL REFLECTION QUESTIONS

- What are your initial responses to this situation?
- What are some strategies for Sally?
- How might Sally proceed in this situation? What are the key considerations?
- What might be other considerations when viewing this case study?

Case study 1.4: Allied health focus

Brian's story

Brian is a second year allied health student who is in his second week of a five-week placement in a regional city hospital. Brian attended a professional development (PD) session presented by an Aboriginal Community Liaison Officer (ACLO) at the start of his placement. The ACLO mentioned that it should be everyone's business who works at the hospital to make sure that the hospital is culturally safe for all clients accessing the services. Since this PD session, Brian has started to reflect on his role as an allied health professional in ensuring that the allied health department is a culturally safe environment for the clients accessing the services. Brian is unsure if the allied health department is culturally safe for the clients as he reflects on a subject that was delivered in his first year at university that spoke of Indigenous clients not being comfortable or safe accessing mainstream health organisations. Brian decides to speak with his supervisor regarding the questions he has.

CRITICAL REFLECTION QUESTIONS

- What are your initial responses to this situation?
- How might Brian proceed in this situation? What key practice considerations arise?
- What might be other considerations when viewing this case study?

Working towards a reconciliation framework

'Reconciliation' is a term that means something different to each individual. As defined by the *Oxford Dictionary of English* (Stevenson, 2017), it is the act of bringing together. Many groups within Australia have a unique and individual focus on reconciliation in regard to Australian people. Key bodies such as the Council for Aboriginal Reconciliation (2000) and Reconciliation Australia (2016, 2017a) all have slightly differing definitions and approaches to reconciliation. Some scholars claim that reconciliation has had a lengthy timeline in Australia with initial steps being taken over 25 years ago via political activity around native title and land rights (Reconciliation Australia, 2017a). The Council for Aboriginal Reconciliation (2000), now superseded by Reconciliation Australia, was foundational in building relationships between Aboriginal and Torres Strait Islander peoples and non-Indigenous Australian people. The historic People's Walk for Reconciliation across the Sydney Harbour Bridge in 2000, following the submission of reconciliation recommendations to the Australian Government, has been described as a pinnacle moment in the Council's history with over 250,000 Australians taking part in the walk (Council for Aboriginal Reconciliation, 2000). Reconciliation Australia is a non-government organisation within Australia with a primary aim to provide a framework for organisations to build capacity and respect (Reconciliation Australia, 2017b). Share our Pride (Reconciliation Australia, 2016), funded by Reconciliation Australia, is a website designed to provide initial thoughts about building better relationships with Aboriginal and Torres Strait Islander peoples.

In 2017, Reconciliation Australia focused on a five-step reconciliation action plan. The five steps involve race relations, equality and equity, institutional integrity, unity, and historical acceptance. One government response to this plan was the bipartisan development of the Referendum Council to consult with Aboriginal and Torres Strait Islander communities on meaningful recognition. Constitutional reform was a focus area recommended. While dialogue still continues, preliminary responses to this suggestion were not in favour of constitutional change (Reconciliation Australia, 2017a).

The Australian Health Practitioner Regulation Agency (AHPRA) (2017) and the national professional boards have often taken a combined approach in defining reconciliation. Reconciliation planning began in 2015 with AHPRA initiating discussion between professional bodies. The overall approach was aimed at professional health bodies seeking ways to close the health gap between Aboriginal and Torres Strait Islander peoples and non-Indigenous Australians. While the plan is still in its infancy, we can conclude that health professional boards in Australia deem reconciliation to be a priority.

A small application of reconciliation was adopted in this textbook. As discussed in the introduction, the development of this textbook involved both an author who identified as Aboriginal and/or Torres Strait Islander and non-Indigenous writers. The journey of the writing team has had both intrinsic and extrinsic opportunities in bringing together health professionals.

Conclusion

The future of nursing and allied health professions requires us to respond to and engage with a variety of cultural groups. To ensure that this response to healthcare is safe for practitioners and clients, we need to encourage all professions to be on a pathway to Indigenous Australian cultural competence. This chapter has provided an exploration of the role of Indigenous Australian cultural competence as a way of working towards a united and unified Australia.

SUMMARY

Throughout this chapter, you have been encouraged to consider models of cultural competence while exploring ways to develop skills in cultural competence. Indigenous Australian cultural competence is a lifelong journey that requires commitment and a willingness to explore the worldview of others.

Learning concept 1

Identify the importance of Indigenous Australian cultural competence: Indigenous Australian cultural competence is a lifelong journey undertaken by health professionals. Indigenous Australian cultural competence encourages us to consider our own bias, worldview, attitude and beliefs. Studies have revealed that Indigenous Australian people are more likely to access healthcare when communication is respectful, where clinicians have an understanding of Indigenous Australian culture, and where clinicians are able to work towards the development of good relationships that involve Indigenous Australian health workers as a part of the healthcare team. It is important that health professionals have the skills, attitudes and beliefs to ensure this is available within Australian healthcare facilities.

Learning concept 2

Identify the historical context behind Indigenous Australian cultural competence: The term 'cultural competence' first emerged in the 1980s in the USA. It was particularly prevalent with teachers, social workers, and health and welfare workers as they were seeking ways to better meet the needs of multicultural communities. Understanding the history assists us to understand contemporary Indigenous Australian cultural competence.

Learning concept 3

Identify the importance of skills that enable the journey of Indigenous Australian cultural competence: Indigenous Australian cultural competence is a lifelong journey with many skills that may influence the journey of individuals. This text provides examples via five major terms: non-linear learning, culture, worldview, discomfort and critical thinking. These provide context in how you may decide to progress your learning journey.

Learning concept 4

Determine strategies that promote Indigenous Australian cultural competence in practice: Acknowledging the journey as involving the concepts of non-linear learning, culture, worldview, discomfort and critical thinking can assist the development of Indigenous Australian cultural competence.

Learning concept 5

Identify your own professional plan in Indigenous Australian cultural competence:
Developing a professional plan will assist in your application and progression in
Indigenous Australian cultural competence.

REVISION QUESTIONS

1. In your own words, explain why the history of cultural competence is important
   to understand.
2. Explore why Indigenous Australian cultural competence requires health
   professionals to be reflective practitioners.
3. Consider your profession and the skills required to be a culturally responsive
   practitioner.
4. Consider how you would contribute to your personal and professional journey in
   Indigenous Australian cultural competence. Develop your own professional plan.
5. Consider Reconciliation Australia's five-step action plan. Review each criterion
   and make suggestions on how you can personally and professionally contribute
   to reconciliation within Australia.

FURTHER READINGS/ADDITIONAL RESOURCES

DiAngelo, R. (2011). White fragility. *International Journal of Critical Pedagogy*, *3*(3), 54-70.

Pattison-Meek, J., & Kovalchuk, S. (2014). Is everyone really equal? An introduction to key
concepts in social justice education. *Journal of Peace Education*, *11*(2), 246-248. doi:10.1080/
17400201.2014.913352

REFERENCES

Australian Bureau of Statistics. (2012). *Australian demographic statistics*. Australian Institute of
Health and Welfare. Canberra: ABS.

Australian Bureau of Statistics. (2015). *Australian demographic statistics*. Australian Institute of
Health and Welfare. Canberra: ABS.

Australian Health Practitioner Regulation Agency (AHPRA). (2017). Australian Health
Practitioner Regulation Agency. Retrieved from https://www.ahpra.gov.au/

Australian Institute of Health and Welfare. (2014). Mortality and life expectancy of
Indigenous Australians: 2008 to 2012. Canberra: AIHW Cat. no. IHW 140.

Australian Institute of Health and Welfare. (2016). 25 years of health expenditure
in Australia: 1989–90 to 2013–14. *Health and Welfare Expenditure Series, No. 56.*
Canberra: AIHW Cat. no. HWE 66.

Australian Nursing & Midwifery Accreditation Council. (2015). *National guidelines for the accreditation of nursing and midwifery programs leading to registration and endorsement in Australia*. Canberra: ANMAC.

Best, O., & Fredericks, B. (Eds.) (2014). *Yatdjuligin: Aboriginal and Torres Strait Islander nursing and midwifery care*. Port Melbourne: Cambridge University Press.

Betancourt, J. R. (2003). Cross-cultural medical education: Conceptual approaches and frameworks for evaluation. *Academic Medicine, 78*(6), 560-569.

Betancourt, J. R., Green, A. R., & Carrillo, J. E. (2002). *Cultural competence in health care: Emerging frameworks and practical approaches* (Vol. 576). New York, NY: Commonwealth Fund, Quality of Care for Underserved Populations.

Biles, J. M. (2017). *Undergraduate nursing and Indigenous Australian cultural competence: The lived experience of students* (unpublished doctoral thesis). Charles Sturt University, Australia.

Biles, J., Coyle, J., Bernoth, M., & Hill, B. (2016). I am looking for my truth: A hermeneutic phenomenological study focusing on undergraduate nursing students' journeys in Indigenous Australian cultural competence. *Journal of Australian Indigenous Issues, 19*(1-2), 161-175.

Boler, M. (2000). An epoch of difference: Hearing voices in the nineties. *Educational Theory, 50*(3), 357-381. doi:10.1111/j.1741-5446.2000.00357.

Brach, C., & Fraser, I. (2000). Can cultural competency reduce racial and ethnic health disparities? A review and conceptual model. *Medical Care Research and Review, 57*(2), 181-217.

Campinha-Bacote, J. (2002). The process of cultural competence in the delivery of healthcare services: A model of care. *Journal of Transcultural Nursing, 13*(3), 181.

Clifford, A., McCalman, J., Bainbridge, R., & Tsey, K. (2015). Interventions to improve cultural competency in health care for Indigenous peoples of Australia, New Zealand, Canada and the USA: A systematic review. *International Journal for Quality in Health Care, 27*(2), 89-98. doi:10.1093/intqhc/mzv010

Commonwealth of Australia. (2013). *National Aboriginal and Torres Strait Islander Health Plan 2013–2023*. Canberra: Commonwealth of Australia.

Commonwealth of Australia. (2016). *Aboriginal and Torres Strait Islander Health Curriculum Framework*. Canberra: Commonwealth of Australia.

Congress of Aboriginal and Torres Strait Islander Nurses and Midwives (CATSINaM). (2017). *The Nursing and Midwifery Aboriginal and Torres Strait Islander Health Curriculum Framework* (Version 1.0), pp. 11-12. Canberra: CATSINaM.

Congress of Aboriginal and Torres Strait Islander Nurses and Midwives (CATSINaM). (2018). *Position statement: Embedding cultural safety across Australian nursing and midwifery*. Canberra: CATSINaM.

Cottrell, S. (2017). *Critical thinking skills*. New York: Palgrave. doi:10.1057/978-1-137-55052-1

Council for Aboriginal Reconciliation. (2000). *Sustaining the reconciliation process*. Canberra: Australian Government Publishing Service.

Council of Australian Governments (COAG) Reform Council. (2010). *National Indigenous Reform Agreement: Baseline Performance Report for 2008–09*. Sydney: Council of Australian Governments (COAG) Reform Council.

Cross, T., Bazron, B., Dennis, K. W., & Isaacs, M. R. (1989). *Towards a culturally competent system of care*. Vol 1. Washington, DC: Child and Adolescent Service System Program Technical Assistance Center.

Durey, A., Thompson, S. C., & Wood, M. (2011). Time to bring down the twin towers in poor Aboriginal hospital care: Addressing institutionalised racism and misunderstandings in communication. *Internal Medicine Journal, 42*(1), 17-22. doi:10.1111/j.1445-5994.2011.02628.x

Eckermann, A., Dowd, T., Chong, E., Nixon, L., Gray, R., & Johnson, S. (2006). *Binan Goonj: Bridging cultures in Aboriginal health* (2nd ed.). Sydney: Churchill Livingstone Elsevier.

Facione, P. A., & Facione, N. C. (2013). Critical thinking for life. *Inquiry: Critical Thinking Across the Disciplines, 28*(1), 5-25. doi:10.5840/inquiryct20132812

Grote, E. (2008). *Principles and practices of cultural competency: A review of the literature*. Canberra: Indigenous Higher Education Advisory Council (IHEAC) and Department of Education, Employment and Workplace Relations.

Hains, A. H., Lynch, E. W., & Winton, P. J. (2000). *Moving towards cross-cultural competence in lifelong personnel development: A review of the literature*. Culturally & Linguistically Appropriate Services. Early Childhood Research Institute on Culturally, Linguistically Appropriate Services. University of Illinois: Urbana-Champaign.

Health Workforce Australia. (2011). *Growing our future: Final report of the Aboriginal and Torres Strait Islander Health Worker Project*. Adelaide: Health Workforce Australia.

Humphery, K. (2000). *Indigenous health and western research*. Discussion Paper No. 2. Melbourne: VicHealth Koori Health Research & Community Development Unit, University of Melbourne.

Hunt, L., Ramjan, L., McDonald, G., Koch, J., Baird, D., & Salamonson, Y. (2015). Nursing students' perspectives of the health and healthcare issues of Australian Indigenous people. *Nurse Education Today, 35*(3), 461-467.

Indigenous Allied Health Australia (IAHA). (2017). *About us*. Retrieved from http://iaha.com.au/about-us/

Indigenous Higher Education Advisory Council (IHEAC). (2007). *Ngapartji-Ngapartji yerra: Stronger futures. Report of the 3rd annual IHEAC conference*. Adelaide: IHEAC. Retrieved from https://trove.nla.gov.au/work/184460021?selectedversion=NBD44294072

Inter-Agency Support Group on Indigenous Peoples' Issues. (2014). *The Health of Indigenous people*. Thematic paper towards the preparation of the 2014 World Conference on Indigenous Peoples. United Nations. Retrieved from http://www.un.org/en/ga/president/68/pdf/wcip/IASG%20Thematic%20Paper%20-%20Health%20-%20rev1.pdf

Jayatilleke, N., & Mackie, A. (2013). Reflection as part of continuous professional development for public health professionals: A literature review. *Journal of Public Health, 35*(2), 308-312. https://doi.org/10.1093/pubmed/fds083

Jenkins, H. (2006). *Convergence culture: Where old and new media collide*. New York: New York University Press.

Kaddoura, M., Van-Dyke, O., & Yang, Q. (2016). Impact of a concept map teaching approach on nursing students' critical thinking skills. *Nursing & Health Sciences, 18*(3), 350-354. doi:10.1111/nhs.12277

Kidd, M. R., Watts, I. T., & Saltman, D. C. (2008). Primary health care reform: Equity is the key. *Medical Journal of Australia*, *189*(4), 221-222.

Larson, A., Gillies, M., Howard, P. J., & Coffin, J. (2007). It's enough to make you sick: The impact of racism on the health of Aboriginal Australians. *Australian and New Zealand Journal of Public Health*, *31*(4), 322-329.

Leininger, M. (1975). Teaching transcultural nursing to transform nursing for the 21st century. *Journal of Transcultural Nursing*, *6*(2), 2-3. doi:10.1177/104365969500600201

Leininger, M. (2002). Culture care assessment for congruent competency practices. In M. M. Leininger & M. R. McFarland (Eds.), *Transcultural nursing: Concepts, theories, research & practice* (3rd ed., pp. 117-144). New York, NY: McGraw-Hill.

Maher, P. (2013). A review of 'traditional' Aboriginal health beliefs. *Australian Journal of Rural Health*, *7*(4), 229-236. doi:10.1046/j.1440-1584.1999.00264.x

McRae, M., Taylor, S. J., Swain, L., & Sheldrake, C. (2008). Evaluation of a pharmacist-led, medicines education program for Aboriginal health workers. *Rural Remote Health*, *8*(4), 946.

Merriam-Webster. (2017). Discomfort. *Webster's dictionary for students* (5th ed.). Springfield: Merriam-Webster.

Mezirow, J. (1981). A critical theory of adult learning and education. *Adult Education, 32*, 3-24.

Mezirow, J. (2010). Learning as transformation: Critical perspectives on a theory in progress. *Choice Reviews Online*, *39*(03), 39-1707. doi:10.5860/choice.39-1707

Mooney, N. B., Bauman, A., Westwood, B., Kelaher, B., Tibben, B., & Jalaludin, B. (2005). A quantitative evaluation of Aboriginal cultural awareness training in an urban health service. *Aboriginal and Islander Health Worker Journal*, *29*(4), 23-30.

National Health and Medical Research Council (NHMRC). (2005). *Cultural competency in health: A guide for policy, partnerships and participation*. Australian Government Canberra: NHMRC. Retrieved from https://www.nhmrc.gov.au/_files_nhmrc/publications/attachments/hp19.pdf

Nurses and Midwifery Board of Australia. (2016). *Registered nurses standards of practice*. Retrieved 20 November 2018 from: https://www.nursingmidwiferyboard.gov.au/Codes-Guidelines-Statements/Professional-standards/registered-nurse-standards-for-practice.aspx

Paul, D., Carr, S., & Milroy, H. (2006). Making a difference: The early impact of an Aboriginal health undergraduate medical curriculum. *Medical Journal of Australia*, *184*, 522-525.

Payne, G., & Payne, J. (2004). *Key concepts in social research*. London: SAGE Publications. doi:10.4135/9781849209397

Purnell, L. D., & Paulanka, B. J. (2003). The Purnell model for cultural competence. In L. Purnell & B. Paulanka (Eds.), *Transcultural health care: A culturally competent approach* (2nd ed., pp. 8-39). Philadelphia: Davis.

Ramsden, I. (1990). *Cultural safety and nursing education in Aotearoa and Te Waipounamu*. PhD thesis. Wellington: Victoria University.

Ranzijn, R., McConnochie, K. R., & Nolan, W. (2009). *Psychology and Indigenous Australians: Foundations of cultural competence*. Australia: Palgrave Macmillan.

Ranzijn, R., McConnochie, K., Day, A., Nolan, W., & Wharton, M. (2008). Towards cultural competence: Australian Indigenous content in undergraduate psychology. *Australian Psychologist*, *43*(2), 132-139.

Reconciliation Australia (2016). People. Stories of success to inspire, encourage and share best practice. *Share Our Pride.* Retrieved from shareourpride.reconciliation.org.au/resource_sections/success-stories/

Reconciliation Australia. (2017a). Building relationships for change between Aboriginal and Torres Strait Islander peoples and other Australians. Retrieved from http://www.reconciliation.org.au

Reconciliation Australia (2017b). What is a RAP. *Reconciliation Action Plans (RAP).* Retrieved from https://www.reconciliation.org.au/reconciliation-action-plans/

Si, D., Bailie, R., Togni, S., Abbs, P., & Robinson, G. W. (2006). Aboriginal health workers and diabetes care in remote community health centres: A mixed method analysis. *Medical Journal of Australia*, *185*(1), 40.

Stevenson, A. (Ed.). (2017). Reconciliation. *Oxford Dictionary of English* (3rd ed.). Oxford: Oxford University Press.

Taylor, K., Thompson, S., & Davis, R. (2010). Delivering culturally appropriate residential rehabilitation for urban Indigenous Australians: A review of the challenges and opportunities. *Australian and New Zealand Journal of Public Health*, *34*(S1), S36-S40. doi:10.1111/j.1753-6405.2010.00551.x

Thomson, N., MacRae, A., Burns, J., Catto, M., Debuyst, O., Krom, I., ... Urquhart, B. (2010). *Overview of Australian Indigenous health status, April 2010.* Perth: Australian Indigenous HealthInfoNet.

Truong, M., Paradies, Y., & Priest, N. (2014). Interventions to improve cultural competency in healthcare: A systematic review of reviews. *BMC Health Services Research*, *14*(1). doi:10.1186/1472-6963-14-99

Underhill, J. (2009). *Humboldt, worldview and language.* Edinburgh: Edinburgh University Press.

Wells, M. (2000). Beyond cultural competence: A model for individual and institutional cultural development. *Journal of Community Health Nursing*, *17*, 189-199.

Young, I. M. (2000). Five faces of oppression. In M. Adams, W. J. Blumenfeld, R. Castaneda, H. Hackman, M. Peters, & X. Zuniga (Eds.), *Reading for diversity and social justice: An anthology on racism, anti-semitism, sexism, heterosexism, ableism and classism* (pp. 35-49). New York: Routledge.

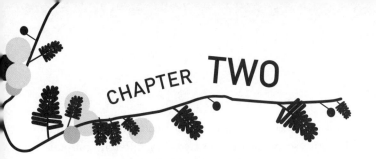

CHAPTER **TWO**

Exploration of history, culture, cultural bias, race and racism

Simone Gray, Brett Biles and Jessica Biles

LEARNING CONCEPTS

Studying this chapter should enable you to:

1. identify the importance of history in relation to Aboriginal and Torres Strait Islander peoples' health.
2. identify the meaning behind race.
3. identify and start to understand what constitutes racism and its impact on individuals and communities.
4. determine how we can consider our own racial background and influences.
5. conclude how as health practitioners we can consider history, race and racism.

KEY TERMS

ethnocentrism

history

privilege

race

racism

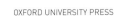

Introduction

Throughout this chapter you will be asked to reflect on your cultural background and consider the impacts of the intersections between two very different cultural groups. You will also consider how **history** can explain the present, particularly within Aboriginal and Torres Strait Islander peoples' cultures due to the cultural transmission of information through generations (Edwards, 1998, p. 23).

history Not a series of agreed facts but something open to interpretation and argument.

History, colonisation and the links to health

Immediately after the arrival of British people to Australia, the health status of Aboriginal and Torres Strait Islander peoples started to decline for a number of important reasons that still impact healthcare today. In particular, introduced disease, dispossession of lands (and therefore access to food sources and medicines), changes in diet due to the introduction of non-traditional (European) foods, and psychological trauma were major contributors (Ranzijn, McConnochie & Nolan, 2009).

Aboriginal and Torres Strait Islander peoples had interacted over many years with foreigners—the French and Dutch visited the shores in the seventeenth century, and the Macassans (from modern-day Sulawesi, Indonesia) were regular trading partners with the Aboriginal people in the north of the country (Clark & May, 2013). It wasn't until the decision to permanently establish a colony in New South Wales that the lives of Aboriginal and Torres Strait Islander peoples were to change remarkably and forever. Early observations by James Cook and Joseph Banks had noted a few inhabitants along the coast, but they assumed there would be even fewer inland. Based on this assumption, Cook declared the land along the east coast of Australia as British (Johnston, 1991). This was the earliest display of ethnocentrism, although it was not perceived that way at the time.

ethnocentrism The lens through which one views the world being dominated by a reflection of people's perceptions (Matsumoto & Juang, 2004).

Ethnocentrism has been defined by Matsumoto and Juang (2004) as something everyone is ingrained with as a result of growing up in specific cultural circumstances, whereby the lens through which they view the world is dominated by a reflection of people's perceptions. It is neither right nor wrong; however, the outcome can be divisiveness due to viewing the world as 'us' versus 'them', thereby judging a particular cultural group. In Australia, this was referred to as 'the Aboriginal problem' (Ellinghaus, 2003). The most important example that still underpins mainstream Australian perceptions of land ownership began with the declaration of 'terra nullius', whereby Aboriginal and Torres Strait Islander peoples were discounted from having property rights or ownership. Thus the disintegration of Indigenous cultures began. Despite the fact that Governor Arthur Phillip came with instructions in 1788 to 'conciliate

[Indigenous peoples'] affections, and to enjoin all subjects to live in amity and kindness with them' (Watson, 1914–1925, p. 12), this did not occur.

Clarke (2008) has recorded some of the history of early settlers utilising the environmental knowledge of the locals, who understood seasonal changes and knew where to find food, which plants were unsafe unless prepared, and how to obtain resources. The knowledge of preparation, which sometimes took days of complicated processing, allowed the continued use of thousands of years of trial and error (Clarke, 2008). A range of meetings occurred between the Eora people and the convicts and soldiers in the first years of the colony. Some encounters were friendly ones of mutual curiosity. Others contained elements of mistrust and violence.

Health and colonisation

Pharmacology was an intrinsic part of Aboriginal and Torres Strait Islander peoples' worldview. Clarke (2008, p. 37) states:

> In Aboriginal cultures, sickness was often attributed to such things as sorcery, breaches of religious sanctions and rules of behaviour, intrusions of spirits and disease-objects, or loss of a person's soul. Cases of swift and inexplicable onset of deadly illness were attributed to supernatural causes.

He also details cases from early accounts of Aboriginal healers attempting to cure people through processes similar to those employed by the Ngangkari (discussed later in this chapter). The appropriation of this knowledge is thought to have contributed to the survival of members of the colony and frontier, providing sources of food, beverages and medicine (Clarke, 2008, p. 41).

Pre-contact Indigenous life included a daily conversation about what was to be resourced by whom and where, based on kinship and totemic responsibilities. The size of the family group depended on their location and the resources available, particularly water (Fryer-Smith, 2008, 2:3; Burden, cited in Bourke, Bourke & Edwards, 1994, p. 192). The resources available meant that animals and plants provided a balanced, nutritious diet that was high in protein with little fat, sugar or salt (Bourke, Bourke & Edwards, 1994, p. 192).

Preparation of food could be easy or hard, and was based on planning the whole sequence, from killing or collecting/digging to cooking. Knowledge of food preparation included resources for food that could not be carried, and knowing what was a restricted food—due to cultural sustainability of taboo foods for people with a certain health condition or in a particular age group or gender (Berndt & Berndt, 1978, p. 47).

To Warlpiri woman Molly Nungarrayi, health meant people looking after each other:

> In the olden days they looked after each other, in the olden time. Poor things, the old people—grandmothers, grandfathers, fathers and mothers—used to look

> after each other ... The people looked after a kinsman until he grew older and
> older and became sick and tired and passed away ... They used to get firewood
> for the old people and make windbreaks and humpies in case it rained ... When
> grandma was sick her husband found bush medicine for her.
>
> Vaarzon-Morel (1995, p. 14)

The complex systems in place and the connection to land meant overall health and wellbeing was intricately enmeshed with totemic responsibilities, and it has been revealed in recent publications and research that the 'hunter-gatherer' title does not articulate the complexity of everyday life (Pascoe, 2014).

Movement was an integral part of lifestyle and it left time for teaching younger generations and recreational play. Games were part of every group's lifestyle (Wheatley, 2011). It was a lifestyle based on the search for and storage of water; on food and medicine; and on reciprocity and collectivism. Keeping a hold on these cultural practices and values was attempted on pastoral stations where people were working on or near their traditional lands; however, the poor diet had an impact on short- and long-term health. Conditions on reserves and missions were also poor, with little thought given to healthcare, fresh water or sanitation needs (Reid & Trompf, 1991, p. 12).

Traditional medicine

The healers in the Anangu language group, who speak and come from the Western Desert, are called 'Ngangkari'. They are men, women and children who have been trained in special knowledges dating back thousands of years. Their cultural knowledge is wholly derived from the Dreaming Law (Ngaanyatjarra Pitjantjatjara Yankunytjatjara Women's Council Aboriginal Corporation, 2013); that is, the knowledge passed onto people from their spirit Ancestors. This work has not ceased thanks to dedicated people. Ngangkari have recently published information and are working in hospitals and with Western healthcare professionals to assist in healing patents who require cultural healing.

> Everyone was healthy because of Ngangkari. Ngangkari would arrive quickly
> when summoned to a sick child ... Ngangkari are skilled at recognising and
> banishing mamu, away from the home wiltja [shelter]. Mamu are harmful spirit
> beings—a dangerous spirit force or energy.
>
> Ngaanyatjarra Pitjantjatjara Yankunytjatjara Women's Council Aboriginal
> Corporation (2013, p. 16)

Sickness and disease

Following contact with Europeans, Aboriginal and Torres Strait Islander peoples were exposed to diseases they had never before encountered. It was written at the time of the first encounters that the health of Aboriginal and Torres Strait Islander peoples was evident: 'We saw them in considerable numbers, and they appeared to us to be a very lively and inquisitive race; they are a straight, thin but well made people, rather small in their limbs, but very active' (Captain John Hunter, 1793, cited in Gilchrist & Murray, 1968, p. 14).

Introduced diseases included influenza, pneumonia, typhoid fever, measles, smallpox, chickenpox, whooping cough, mumps, scarlet fever, diphtheria, tuberculosis, gonorrhoea and various venereal diseases (Reid & Trompf, 1991, p. 5). It is important to note that although some of these were known to affect children in Europe, Aboriginal and Torres Strait Islander populations were impacted at all ages; and due to the nature of the diseases, all members of a family or community could fall ill at the same time, meaning that no one was available to care for them, which increased the fatality rate (Reid & Trompf, 1991, p. 6).

Irish (2017) explains that when the Sydney smallpox epidemic of 1789 was over, the surviving Aboriginal groups of the Sydney area had to regroup as the settlement began to grow with more ships arriving. Many Elders and women had died, straining knowledge transmission and affecting reproduction, underpinned by events and practices that were unexplainable as 'their core beliefs were shaken' (Irish, 2017, p. 22). Regroup they did, incorporating new British knowledge into cultural practices, staying on the land by seeking employment in town, and continuing the cultural practice of fishing, which allowed self-sufficiency (Irish, 2017, p. 36).

Health and the land

Aboriginal and Torres Strait Islander peoples are now regarded as highly efficient environmental managers, although this management had always been an integrated and well-established pattern of caring for the earth as understood in Dreaming Law (Gammage, 2011; Pascoe, 2014). For Aboriginal and Torres Strait Islander peoples, the pattern of enforced removal from the land and the subsequent destruction of the carefully managed environment meant that spiritual, psychological and physical health was radically altered (Ranzijn et al., 2009).

In 1829 on the other side of the continent (known as Western Australia), the rugged bushland, swamps and small lakes that enabled local people to survive were soon to be invaded (Adams, 2009). A freshwater source by the sea was vital, and after establishing a pattern of movement around it, the settlers decided to claim the spot for themselves. The settlers then built the Roundhouse Gaol, which was later the place from which men from all over Western Australia were deported to die on Rottnest Island (Adams, 2009).

Evidence collected by Gammage (2011) from across Australia suggests three key ideas about land management prior to European arrival: that nearly three-quarters of native plants required or tolerated fire, and management of that needed to be managed carefully and locally; that this allowed management of grazing fauna; and that this was achievable by following Law, an underpinning 'ecological philosophy' that was imperative to survival (Gammage, 2011, pp. 1–2). This knowledge is now being revitalised among communities and is considered a highly complex technique by twenty-first-century ecological managers. One contemporary example is the Fire Management Plan in the Australian Capital Territory (Lowry, 2016).

Violence

In New South Wales, Pemulwuy and other warriors took it upon themselves to engage in open and guerrilla warfare, but were overpowered by the number of British troops and guns (Broome, 2010). The dispossession of Aboriginal and Torres Strait Islander peoples from their lands was violent and included shootings, rape, capture, kidnapping and poisoning of waterholes. The rate of colonisation was different in each colony, but across the country those who would not relinquish their sovereignty were brutally punished (Broome, 2010). Disciplining people by use of physical force, such as whippings and beatings, was common and reinforced by ethnocentric ideas (Reid & Trompf, 1991, p. 9).

This period of time was known as 'the frontier' (Reynolds, 1987) The frontier was characterised by a scarcity of resources and there are many documented cases where the only fresh waterholes were deliberately poisoned by white settlers to eradicate the use of the water by Aboriginal and Torres Strait Islander peoples (Lydon, 1996). In other cases, food was poisoned and left out. Massacres of people continued from colonisation through to the 1920s, and the relocation of healthy people into settlements (reserves or missions) with unhygienic conditions contributed to the conflicting policy directions towards Aboriginal and Torres Strait Islander peoples (Reid & Trompf, 1991). Large-scale killings came to an end in some places as Aboriginal and Torres Strait Islander people moved onto pastoral stations to endeavour to work to survive. Some were fortunate that they were able to work on traditional lands, thus allowing them to attempt to maintain cultural practices (Broome, 2010).

Influence of racial thought

The British brought with them an understanding of a hierarchy that placed them at the top (Ardill, 2009). Charles Darwin published *On the Origin of Species* in 1859, outlining the theory of evolution (Darwin, 1859); these ideas were formulated into the concept of 'social Darwinism' and influenced Australian history.

In Australia, Aboriginal and Torres Strait Islander people's bodies and bones were stolen and used in research. Collections are still held in European and Australian museums. Aboriginal and Torres Strait Islander peoples were studied extensively, but always through the prism of British theories and discourses (Burden, 2018)

The concept of race and evolution was later to be used for the classification of Aboriginal people, and the introduction of the terms 'half-caste', 'full-bloods' and 'quadroons' was to play a major role in the future treatment of Aboriginal and Torres Strait Islander peoples. Eckermann, Dowd, Chong, Nixon, Gray and Johnson (2010, p. 9) explain that the rise of science combined with the Industrial Revolution presented what is now referred to as 'scientific racism', whereby Aboriginal people were considered to be locked in the Stone Age; to survive by instinct not intellect; to have only basic cultural systems; and to be childlike and therefore unpredictable. Together these beliefs created a British understanding of 'Aboriginality'.

Case study 2.1: General healthcare

Denise's story

Denise is a woman of Anglo heritage who admits herself to the birthing room at her local hospital. She gives birth to a son with blonde hair and blue eyes. Her partner attends the birth and they proceed to discuss the two options to name their son—Connor or Djarra. The midwife and doctor exchange puzzled looks, so the mother explains that her partner is of Aboriginal heritage and therefore so is their son. They decide on the name Djarra and then have to explain its origins from a family language dictionary. A day later, after receiving the paperwork to be released to go home, Denise realises that the form has changed. She had ticked the box stating that her son was to identify as Aboriginal, but the tick has been removed. She queries the nursing staff, whose response is that they thought she had made a mistake. Denise is embarrassed and angry.

CRITICAL REFLECTION QUESTIONS

- Why do you think Denise felt this way?
- What message does this send to the family from the nursing staff?
- Thinking about the power relations, how do you think you would have approached the identity of the child?

Case study 2.2: Allied health focus

Sophie's story

Sophie is studying podiatry and has read the history of racial ideology and its impacts on Aboriginal and Torres Strait Islander peoples. She is appalled that she has been unaware of the impacts on health outcomes. She discusses it with

(Continued)

a colleague, Alison, who is studying nutrition. Alison is aware of policies that had separated Aboriginal and Torres Strait Islander peoples from mainstream society, but was unaware of Aboriginal and Torres Strait Islander peoples' perspectives on health and wellbeing. They both decide that their understanding of Aboriginal and Torres Strait Islander peoples' knowledges about health and wellbeing is inadequate. They realise that they have not considered the fact that 50,000 years of health and wellbeing has been largely ignored by their professions.

CRITICAL REFLECTION QUESTIONS

- Should Sophie and Alison undertake further research? If so, in what areas?
- Should they go to an Indigenous person and ask for more information?
- How would undertaking further research help them to provide better healthcare outcomes for Aboriginal and Torres Strait Islander peoples?

Policy decisions and their impact on health

In the late 1800s, the various Australian colonies started to implement legislation or other mechanisms. This involved the development of policies that were detrimental to the health of Aboriginal and Torres Strait Islander peoples, impacting physical, cultural, spiritual and mental health (Sherwood, 2013).

Reid and Trompf (1991) believe that one of the reasons for moving people onto reserves and Christian missions was to remove people from land to prevent hunting and gathering, as the land had been prioritised to support European-style agriculture and grazing. Aboriginal and Torres Strait Islander peoples then became reliant on a poor diet as the rations tended to be 'cheap, portable and non-perishable' (p. 11). The fact that Aboriginal and Torres Strait Islander peoples had their own complex resource management systems—including eel farming, cultivation of yams and many other methods of producing sustainable resources, including nourishing food—was ignored, undervalued or unknown to those in authority (Pascoe, 2014).

Conditions on reserves and missions were in some cases appalling, with little to no access to sanitation systems and fresh water (Reid & Trompf, 1991), while housing infrastructure continued to be a low priority, especially in rural and remote areas. Further, the active segregation of Aboriginal and Torres Strait Islander peoples from mainstream society meant that any health facilities were poorly maintained, with staff on the missions and reserves having little to no medical experience or training, and no knowledge of the holistic worldview of health and wellbeing held by Aboriginal and

Torres Strait Islander peoples (Franklin & White, pp. 10–18, in Reid & Trompf, 1991). The overcrowded and sedentary living conditions affected adults in particular as their daily routines were no longer available (Burden, in Bourke, Bourke & Edwards, p. 195).

Conditions on pastoral stations were not any better, as Aboriginal men and women were paid far less than other workers, were similarly housed in bare conditions and were reliant on rations (Broome, 2010). Reid and Trompf (1991, pp. 16–18) cite research undertaken from the 1940s to 1960s that raised concerns regarding the treatment and conditions of Aboriginal and Torres Strait Islander people on stations. These included the high mortality and morbidity rates of children and the refusal by Aboriginal and Torres Strait Islander peoples to rear their children as slaves.

Uncle Max Dulumunmun Harrison (2009) explained that traditional food was meant to maintain health and that 'good Samaritans' looking at Aboriginal people living in missions decided that they were underfed and undernourished on the basis of their slim, slender and muscular builds from natural diets: 'And that's when the sugars and flours came into our diet ... we became disconnected from the Earth Mother for nutrition, and dependent on the white man's tucker' (Harrison, 2009, p. 146).

Harrison also believes that clothes, coats and blankets caused people's immune systems to be affected: 'Our bodies were used to the nakedness, used to the cold and every time we swam in Gadu we would ingest salt down the throat and nose, and that salt would help build up immunity against our winter ailments' (Harrison, 2009, p. 149).

Protection

Around the time the British overturned the practice of slavery within its jurisdictions in 1833, a British Committee of the Parliament took evidence from witnesses while investigating the conditions of Aboriginal and Torres Strait Islander peoples. Governor Arthur described the failed attempt in Tasmania to co-exist (Reynolds, 1987). The Committee appointed Protectors for Aboriginal and Torres Strait Islander peoples, which led to the grouping of people in reserves and missions. Those on reserves were able to maintain some cultural traditions, but often would leave when rations became scarce. Wherever they were, authorities were removing children and taking them from their families (Broome, 2010, p. 53).

The National Inquiry into the Separation of Aboriginal and Torres Strait Islander Children from their Families, otherwise known as the *Bringing Them Home* report (Wilson & Australian Human Rights and Equal Opportunity Commission, 1997), estimated that up to 100,000 children were removed by 'compulsion, duress or undue influence' (p. 5). Impacts on health were enormous, with most suffering psychological harm. The report also details sexual and physical abuse in many cases, and the long-lasting impacts involving many facets of people's lives.

Government policy at the state and territory level largely ignored the issue of Aboriginal and Torres Strait Islander peoples' health. The belief in mainstream society, fostered by social Darwinism in the 1880s, was that 'full-blooded' Aboriginal people would die out, as the 'race' was doomed to extinction, and the White Australia policy formed in 1901 reconfirmed the underpinning idea that Australia was to be a 'white' country (Broome, 2010, p. 198), albeit with some minorities who had already arrived. Protection legislation allowed for more control at each amendment. The 1915 amendment removed the necessity for authorities to seek permission from Aborigines Protection Boards to remove children. Legislation ultimately controlled every facet of Aboriginal and Torres Strait Islander peoples' lives (Ranzijn et al., 2009, p. 95).

By the 1930s, activists began to complain about the removal of children and the fact that people were being segregated. Interestingly, the 1930s also saw work by anthropologists trying to add to the understanding of Indigenous people; in particular, Dr Phyllis Kaberry (1939) investigated the role and 'place' of Aboriginal women in the Kimberley. She noted that:

> More positively we can say that their way of life would seem to contribute to their health, endow them with a store of vitality and physical fitness which enable them to grapple with the exacting conditions of environment and climate.
>
> Kaberry (1939, p. 35)

The Australian Aborigines Progressive Association, formed in 1937 under the leadership of Fred Maynard, fought for, among other issues, the end to the forced removal of children from their families, and the end of exploitation of Aboriginal and Torres Strait Islander women by non-Indigenous men (Maynard, 2007).

The Australian Aborigines' League, formed by William Cooper and others in 1938, also fought to stop the removal of children (Attwood & Markus, 2004). These organisations paved the way for further activism and acknowledgment of rights and equity, which sparked the successful 'yes' vote in the 1967 referendum. By the 1960s, many Aboriginal and Torres Strait Islander peoples were fighting for rights, including those of families and children (Wilson & Australian Human Rights and Equal Opportunity Commission, 1997, p. 376). Activism allowed for the establishment of the first Aboriginal Medical Service in Redfern, Sydney in 1971.

Despite the efforts of these activist organisations, the Commonwealth and state 'Aboriginal authorities' held a conference in Canberra in 1937 to discuss the 'destiny of the [Aboriginal] race' and again in 1961 when an official definition of 'assimilation' was developed (Hasluck, 1961). Protection had been a means of biological absorption, whereas assimilation focused on cultural absorption requiring all authorities to take 'temporary' and 'special' measures to allow Aboriginal and Torres Strait Islander peoples to 'live as members of a single Australia' and to encourage 'their future social, economic and political advancement' (Hasluck, 1961).

Aboriginal and Torres Strait Islander peoples have been subjected to institutionalised racism, which reflects the attitudes of governments and authorities that historically never took into account Aboriginal and Torres Strait Islander peoples' worldviews (Eckermann et al., 2010). This changed with the establishment of Aboriginal Community Controlled Health Organisations (ACCHPs), discussed in Chapter 3.

Race and racism

As we have previously discussed, human nature stems from history and society. Exploration of the history of ourselves and others is important when we consider and start to understand race and racism. Scholars have argued that multiple factors that result in racism stem from previous acts of power and **privilege** that influence social practice (Foucault, 1980).

The term 'racist' is not a new term. In fact, it originated from Plato and Aristotle's philosophical concept of the Great Chain of Being, which raised our awareness of humanity having a hierarchy (Zalta, 2008). This led to the idea that 'race' was a set of characteristics and achievements that made one superior or inferior, and thus behaviours became 'racist' (Hampton & Toombs, 2013). Today, some understanding of **race** and racism is required by all health professionals due to the power and privilege that we hold when clients are at their most vulnerable. Exploration of self is essential to start to understand how others may see the world. As discussed in Chapter 1, this is a distinct part of the journey of Indigenous Australian cultural competence. Being aware of our own history, race and identity is at the forefront in being able to understand the 'other'. We will explore this further within this chapter.

privilege A special right, advantage or immunity granted or available only to a particular person or group.

race People identified as members of a group because of their physical appearance, culture or ethnic origin—real or supposed.

Racism

Literature on **racism** describes four different forms:

1 *institutional racism*, which involves the incorporation of racist ideals in policies and practices within an organisation
2 *individual racism*, which is the support of racist ideals by individuals and small groups
3 *cultural racism*, which is where the beliefs, ideals and values of a cultural group are seen to be superior to opposing groups
4 *modern racism*, which is the subtle cues and expressions that involve rejection of minority groups (Hampton & Toombs, 2013; Ranzijn, McConnochie, Day, Nolan & Wharton, 2008; Australian Human Rights Commission, 2011).

racism Prejudice, discrimination or antagonism directed against someone of a different race based on the belief that one's own race is superior.

While all definitions of racism are important, institutional and individual racism will be the focus of this text.

Institutional racism is defined as the policies, systems and practices that exclude members of a non-dominant group and thus permeate norms within an institution (Hampton & Toombs, 2013). Individual racism, in the provision of health services, is behaviour that takes on a form of clinical uncertainty within the interaction between client and health professional that can be intentional or unintentional (Larson, Gillies, Howard & Coffin, 2007). Larson et al. further indicated, in a quantitative study, that racism prevents Aboriginal and Torres Strait Islander peoples from regularly accessing healthcare, highlighting the detrimental effects of institutional influence on health. Kleinman, Eisenberg and Good (1978) drew attention to the concept of illness and treatment as being culturally shaped. From this, a link became evident that health providers' responsiveness to cultural differences could lead to improved health outcomes.

The loss, trauma and inhibition in all aspects of Aboriginal and Torres Strait Islander peoples' social, physical and mental life were articulated in the *Bringing Them Home* report (Wilson & Australian Human Rights and Equal Opportunity Commission, 1997). This report was based on the National Inquiry into the Separation of Aboriginal and Torres Strait Islander Children from their Families and details the loss, hardship, struggle and strength of those children who were removed from their families by the Australian government. The report's recommendations highlighted the importance of racial policy and social behaviours in Australia and how they can influence intergenerational health outcomes. This notion is supported by the Australian Bureau of Statistics, which reported, in 2008, that Aboriginal and Torres Strait Islander clients accessing care received care that was neither sensitive to cultural needs nor culturally appropriate (Australian Bureau of Statistics, 2008). Within Australia we have some work to do in this space to ensure that healthcare is accessible for all.

Institutional racism

Institutional racism in healthcare involves systems that oppose or oppress identifiable groups based on race or ethnicity (Durey, Thompson & Wood, 2011). Researchers in Western Australia noted that the prejudice Aboriginal and Torres Strait Islander peoples experience was more than twice that of any other Australian. This occurred for more than 43% of respondents in everyday life situations (Dunn, Forrest, Pe-Pua, Hynes & Maeder-Han, 2009) and particularly when liaising with institutions such as police, education and health, leaving little doubt that institutional racism is evident in Australia (Pedersen, Dudgeon, Watt & Griffiths, 2006). It is argued that in Australian healthcare systems, racism is experienced in facilities that are founded on Western models of care, with minimal diversity in the ethnicity of healthcare professionals (Durey et al., 2011; Williamson & Harrison, 2010). Frameworks aimed at reducing institutional racism have been implemented by healthcare facilities within Australia (Australian Institute of Health and Welfare, 2011).

The *Social Justice Report* (Aboriginal & Torres Strait Islander Social Justice Commissioner, 2005) highlighted the impact of racism not only at an individual level, but also at an institutional level, with Australian mainstream health policy delivery failing to support Aboriginal and Torres Strait Islander peoples. This was cited as the result of a poorly developed health policy framework and strategic direction. Given that the publication *Overview of Australian Indigenous Status* (Thomson et al., 2010) details that Aboriginal and Torres Strait Islander peoples' morbidity and mortality rates are disproportionately high compared with non-Indigenous Australians, the consideration of the health policy framework is important. The need for Australian health systems to respond to all clients in a culturally appropriate fashion is important (Larson et al., 2007). In a report drafted by the United Nations, the issues of racism and discrimination were highlighted as significant barriers for indigenous peoples globally accessing healthcare. This report clearly articulated the lack of cultural sensitivity by health services that inhibits indigenous people from accessing these facilities (United Nations, 2014).

Individual racism

Individual racism in Australia relates to the inherent paternalism that influences the power dynamic in health relationships between client and health professional (Jackson, Brady & Stein, 1999). Coupled with the relative paucity of Aboriginal and Torres Strait Islander staff in positions of influence, this creates a situation where making sustainable cultural and social change within an organisation is challenging (Dollard, Stewart, Fuller & Blue, 2001; Taylor, Thompson & Davis, 2010). Limited knowledge of Aboriginal and Torres Strait Islander peoples' cultures and communities contributes to individual racism within healthcare facilities in Australia (Williamson & Harrison, 2010; Reibel & Walker, 2010; Pedersen et al., 2006), further indicating the need for health workforce training in this space.

IMPLICATIONS FOR NURSING AND ALLIED HEALTH PRACTICE

The Registered Nurse Code of Conduct and the Professional Standards have defined professional conduct and behaviours to ensure that all consumers of healthcare are able to access care. Review these standards.

Similarly, every registered allied health professional must follow their respective code of conduct. Within in each code of conduct, behaviour regarding race, racism and discrimination is mandated. Review your professional code of conduct.

Case study 2.3: General healthcare

Madeleine's story

Madeleine is 10 years old. She has been experiencing some gastro-intestinal upsets and has decided to consult her local GP with her mother Bernadette. Madeleine's usual GP was not available so they accepted an appointment with a

(Continued)

female GP in their usual clinic. The GP was friendly and made some appropriate suggestions related to Madeleine's health complaint. As a referral was being written, the GP noticed that Madeleine identified as Aboriginal. The GP was surprised and stated, 'You don't look Aboriginal—you have fair skin'. This was not unusual in Madeleine's world and she proceeded to explain that Indigeneity is about identity. Madeleine was proud of her ability to explain this and smiled at her mum. The GP didn't comment for a while. She then said, 'Most Aboriginal people have brown skin and a flat nose'. Madeleine's mum Bernadette started to explain the history of the Stolen Generations to the GP, who promptly interrupted and said, 'I had another patient the other day who looked Italian but said they were also Aboriginal'. Madeleine and her mum ended the appointment. Madeleine told her mum that she felt very uncomfortable and didn't want to see that GP again.

CRITICAL REFLECTION QUESTIONS

- What are your initial responses to this situation?
- What key practice considerations arise?
- What might be other considerations if viewing this case through the lens of Aboriginal and Torres Strait Islander peoples' history?
- What implications might this have for Madeleine's long-term health?

Case study 2.4: Allied health focus

Bruce's story

Bruce is an Aboriginal man who suffered a myocardial infarction at the age of 42. After recovering from his stent insertion surgery, Bruce had to attend six weeks of cardiac rehabilitation at his local hospital, with two sessions per week. Bruce was the youngest in the group and often found himself having 'courageous conversations' around race with the other participants, who were at least 20 years older than Bruce. For example, during the morning tea break Bruce was having a cuppa with John. John said, 'Bruce, back when I was a bit younger I knew an Aborigine,' which was then followed by, 'Are there many Aborigines in our town?' Bruce is a community leader and felt that he needed to educate John on appropriate and current terminology. The conversation ended well, but this type of conversation was a common occurrence for Bruce throughout his cardiac rehab.

Bruce approaches you as a health professional and explains how exhausting it is to provide cultural education while completing his cardiac rehab journey.

CRITICAL REFLECTION QUESTIONS

- What are your initial responses to this situation?
- What strategies could you implement to support Bruce's journey?
- What is the risk of not responding to Bruce's concerns?
- Where could you go to seek support in navigating this situation?

Conclusion

The future of nursing and allied health professions will require us to engage with different cultural groups. It is imperative that we are able to understand how historical legacies along with race and racism impact on contemporary health issues. It is also important to understand that racism still exists today and we need to be aware and understand how our privilege can impact on the health requirements of the clients we treat.

SUMMARY

Throughout this chapter, you have been encouraged to reflect on your cultural background and consider the impacts of history, race and racism on two very different cultural groups. You have explored history and considered how the past and present have influenced Aboriginal and Torres Strait Islander peoples' health outcomes.

Learning concept 1

Identify the importance of history in relation to Aboriginal and Torres Strait Islander peoples' health: History can enhance our understanding, providing an important tool for health professionals when working with Aboriginal and Torres Strait Islander peoples.

Learning concept 2

Identify the meaning behind racism: 'Racism' has been defined as prejudice, discrimination or antagonism directed against someone of a different race based on the belief that one's own race is superior. Some understanding of race and racism is required by health professionals. This is due to the power and privilege that we hold when clients are at their most vulnerable.

Learning concept 3

Identify and start to understand what constitutes racism and its impact on individuals and communities: Institutional racism is defined as the policies, systems and practices that exclude members of a non-dominant group and thus permeate norms within an institution. In the provision of health services, individual racism is behaviour that takes on a form of clinical uncertainty within the interaction between client and health professional that can be intentional or unintentional.

Learning concept 4

Determine how we can consider our own racial background and influences: Our own racial background is important to explore so that we can discover the nuances and ways of being that make us unique and thus enable us to understand others.

Learning concept 5

Conclude how as health practitioners we can consider history, race and racism: Health professionals must consider how historical legacies along with race and racism impact on contemporary health issues. It is also important to understand that racism still exists today and we need to be aware and understand how our privilege influences healthcare delivery and healthcare outcomes.

REVISION QUESTIONS

1. Explain how this chapter links to the Australian Registered Nurse Code of Professional Conduct and Code of Ethics in Nursing.
2. In your own words explain what the evidence-based research indicates are the physiological impacts of negative behaviours that are directed towards a person's race.

FURTHER READINGS/ADDITIONAL RESOURCES

Elder, B. (1998). *Blood on the wattle: Massacres and mistreatments of Aboriginal Australians since 1788*. Sydney: New Holland Publishers.

MacDonald, R., & Australian Archives. (1995). *Between two worlds: The Commonwealth government and the removal of Aboriginal children of part descent in the Northern Territory*. Alice Springs: IAD Press.

Presland, G. (2010). *First people: The Eastern Kulin of Melbourne, Port Phillip and Central Victoria*. Museum Victoria.

OXFORD UNIVERSITY PRESS

REFERENCES

Aboriginal & Torres Strait Islander Social Justice Commissioner. (2005). *Social Justice Report*. Canberra, Australia: Human Rights and Equal Opportunity Commission. https://www. humanrights.gov.au/sites/default/files/content/social_justice/sj_report/sjreport05/pdf/ SocialJustice2005.pdf

Adams, S. (2009). *The unforgiving rope: Murder and hanging on Western Australia's frontier*. WA: UWA Publishing.

Ardill, A. (2009). Sociobiology, racism, and Australian colonisation. *Griffith Law Review*, *18*(1), 82-113.

Attwood, B., & Markus, A. (2004). *Thinking black: William Cooper and the Australian Aborigines' League*. [online]. Canberra: Aboriginal Studies Press. https://search-informit-com-au.ezproxy. csu.edu.au/documentSummary;dn=389447139480803;res=IELIND

Australian Bureau of Statistics. (2008). *Experimental life tables for Aboriginal and Torres Strait Islanders Australians, 2005–2007*. Canberra: ABS.

Australian Human Rights Commission. (2011). *Social justice report 2011*. Canberra: Australian Human Rights Commission.

Australian Human Rights Commission. (2016). *All about age discrimination*. Retrieved from http://www.humanrights.gov.au/all-about-age-discrimination

Australian Institute of Health and Welfare. (2011). *The health and welfare of Australia's Aboriginal and Torres Strait Islander people: An overview: 2011*. Canberra: Australian Institute of Health and Welfare.

Berndt, C. H., & Berndt, R. M. (1978). *Pioneers and settlers: the Aboriginal Australians*. Carlton: Pitman Publishing.

Bourke, C. Bourke, E & Edwards, B. (1994). *Aboriginal Australia: An introductory reader in Aboriginal Studies* (2nd ed.). Brisbane: University of Queensland Press.

Broome, R. (2010). *Aboriginal Australians: A history since 1788* (4th ed.). Crows Nest: Allen & Unwin.

Burden, G. (2018). The violent collectors who gathered Indigenous artefacts for the Queensland Museum. *The Conversation*. Retrieved from https://theconversation.com/the-violent-collectors-who-gathered-indigenous-artefacts-for-the-queensland-museum-96119

Burden, J. (1994). Health: An holistic approach (chap. 10). In C. Bourke, E. Bourke & B. Edwards (1994), *Aboriginal Australia: An introductory reader in Aboriginal Studies* (2nd ed.). University of Queensland Press.

Clark, M., & May, S. K. (2013). *Macassan history and heritage journeys, encounters and influences*. Canberra: ANU Press.

Clarke, P. A. (2008). *Aboriginal plant collectors: Botanists and Australian Aboriginal people in the nineteenth century*. Kenthurst NSW: Rosenberg Publishing Pty. Ltd.

Darwin, C. (1859). *On the origin of species*. London: John Murray.

Dollard, J., Stewart, T., Fuller, J., & Blue, I. (2001). Aboriginal health worker status in South Australia. *Aboriginal and Islander Health Worker Journal*, *24*(1), 28.

Dunn, K. M., Forrest, J., Pe-Pua, R., Hynes, M., & Maeder-Han, K. (2009). Cities of race hatred? The spheres of racism and anti-racism in contemporary Australian cities. *Cosmopolitan Civil Societies: An Interdisciplinary Journal*, *1*(1). doi:10.5130/ccs.v1i1.833

Durey, A., Thompson, S. C., & Wood, M. (2011). Time to bring down the twin towers in poor Aboriginal hospital care: Addressing institutionalised racism and misunderstandings in communication. *Intern Med Journal, 42*(1), 17-22. doi:10.1111/j.1445-5994.2011.02628.x

Eckermann, A. K., Dowd, T., Chong, E., Nixon, L., Gray, R., & Johnson, S. (2010). *Binan Goonj: Bridging cultures in Aboriginal health* (3rd ed.). Sydney: Elsevier/Churchill Livingstone.

Edwards, W. H. (1998). *An Introduction to Aboriginal Societies* (2nd ed.). South Melbourne: Cengage Learning Australia Pty Ltd.

Ellinghaus, K. (2003). *Absorbing the 'Aboriginal problem': Controlling interracial marriage in Australia in the late 19th and early 20th centuries.* Canberra: ANU Press. http://press-files.anu.edu.au/downloads/press/p73641/pdf/ch1128.pdf

Foucault, M. (1980). *Power/knowledge: Selected interviews and other writings, 1972–1977.* Oxford: Harvester Press.

Fryer-Smith. (2008). Aboriginal benchbook for Western Australian courts. Retrieved from https://aija.org.au/wp-content/uploads/2017/07/Aboriginal-Benchbook-for-WA-Courts-2nd-Ed.pdf

Gammage, B. (2011). *The biggest estate on earth: How Aborigines made Australia.* Sydney: Allen & Unwin.

Gilchrist, J. T., & Murray, W. J. (Eds.). (1968). Eye-witness: Selected documents from Australia's past. Australia: Rigby Limited.

Hampton, R., & Toombs, M. (Eds.). (2013). *Indigenous Australians and health. The wombat in the room.* Docklands: Oxford University Press Australia/New Zealand.

Harrison, M. D. (2013). *My people's dreaming: An Aboriginal elder speaks on life, land, spirit and forgiveness.* Australia: Harper Collins Publishers.

Hasluck, P. (1961). *The policy of assimilation: Decisions of Commonwealth and state ministers at the Native Welfare Conference, Canberra, January 26th and 27th, 1961.* Canberra: Commonwealth Govt. Printer. Retrieved from https://aiatsis.gov.au/sites/default/files/catalogue_resources/18801.pdf

Irish, P. (2017). *Hidden in plain view: The Aboriginal people of coastal Sydney.* Australia: NewSouth Books.

Jackson, D., Brady, W., & Stein, I. (1999). Towards (re)conciliation: (re)constructing relationships between Indigenous health workers and nurses. *Journal of Advanced Nursing, 29*(1), 97-103.

Johnston, E. (1991). 10.3 The Dispossession of Aboriginal People. *Royal Commission into Aboriginal Deaths in Custody National Report, Vol. 2.* Canberra: Australian Government Publishing Service. http://www.austlii.edu.au/au/other/IndigLRes/rciadic/national/vol2/

Kaberry, P. M. (1939). *Aboriginal woman: Sacred and profane.* London: George Routledge & Sons Ltd.

Kleinman, A., Eisenberg, L., & Good, B. (1978). Culture, illness, and care: clinical lessons from anthropologic and cross-cultural research. Annals of Internal Medicine, 88(2), 251–258.

Larson, A., Gillies, M., Howard, P. J., & Coffin. J. (2007). It's enough to make you sick: The impact of racism on the health of Aboriginal Australians. *Australia and New Zealand Journal of Public Health, 31*(4), 322-329.

Lowry, T. (2016). Indigenous fire practices used in hazard-reduction burns at significant ACT cultural sites. *ABC News*, 1 April 2016. Retrieved from http://www.abc.net.au/news/2016-04-01/indigenous-fire-practices-used-in-hazard-reduction-burns-in-act/7293212

Lydon, J. (1996). 'No moral doubt...': Aboriginal evidence and the Kangaroo Creek poisoning, 1847–1849. *Aboriginal History*, 20(1996), 151-175. http://press-files.anu.edu.au/downloads/press/p72561/pdf/article0714.pdf

Matsumoto, D., & Juang, L. (2004*). Culture and psychology* (3rd ed.). California: Thomson/Wadsworth.

Maynard, J. (2007). *Fight for liberty and freedom: The origins of Australian Aboriginal activism.* Canberra: Aboriginal Studies Press.

Ngaanyatjarra Pitjantjatjara Yankunytjatjara Women's Council Aboriginal Corporation (2013). *Traditional healers of Central Australia: Ngangkari*. Broome: Magabala Books Aboriginal Corporation.

Pascoe, B. (2014). *Dark emu black seeds: Agriculture or accident?* Broome: Magabala Books Aboriginal Corporation.

Pedersen, A., Dudgeon, P., Watt, S., & Griffiths, B. (2006). Attitudes towards Indigenous Australians: The issue of special treatment. *Australian Psychologist*, 41(2), 85-94.

Ranzijin, R., McConnochie, K., Day, A., Nolan, W., & Wharton, M. (2008). Towards cultural competence: Australian Indigenous content in undergraduate psychology. *Australian Psychologist*, 43(2), 132-139.

Ranzijn, R., McConnochie, K., & Nolan, W. (2009). *Psychology and Indigenous Australians: Foundations of Cultural Competence*. South Yarra: Palgrave Macmillan.

Reibel, T., & Walker, R. (2010). Antenatal services for Aboriginal women: The relevance of cultural competence. *Quality in Primary Care*, 18, 65-74.

Reid, R., & Trompf, P. (Eds.). (1991). *The health of Aboriginal Australia.* Marrickville: Harcourt Brace & Company.

Reynolds, H. (1987). *Frontier: Aborigines, settlers and land.* St Leonards: Allen & Unwin.

Sherwood, J. (2013). Colonisation—it's bad for your health: The context of Aboriginal health. *Contemporary Nurse*, 46(1). doi:10.5172/conu.2013.46.1.28

Taylor, K., Thompson, S., & Davis, R. (2010). Delivering culturally appropriate residential rehabilitation for urban Indigenous Australians: A review of the challenges and opportunities. *Australian and New Zealand Journal of Public Health*, 34, S36-S40. doi:10.1111/j.1753-6405.2010.00551.x

Thomson, N., MacRae, A., Burns, J., Catto, M., Debuyst, O., Krom, I., ... Urquhart, B. (2010). *Overview of Australian Indigenous health status, April 2010*. Perth: Australian Indigenous HealthInfoNet.

United Nations. (2014). Secretariat of Permanent Forum on Indigenous Issues. Human Rights Documents Online. doi:10.1163/2210-7975_hrd-4025-0014.

Vaarzon-Morel, P. (Ed.), Nungarrayi, M., & Institute for Aboriginal Development. (1995). *Warlpiri karnta karnta-kurlangu yimi=Warlpiri women's voices: our lives, our history.* Alice Springs: IAD Press.

Watson, F. (1914–1925). *Historical Records of Australia* [online]. Australian Parliamentary Joint Library Committee. https://trove.nla.gov.au/work/17995589

Wheatley, N. (2011). *Playground: Listening to stories from country and from inside the heart.* Crows Nest: Allen & Unwin.

Williamson, M., & Harrison, L. (2010). Providing culturally appropriate care: A literature review. *International Journal of Nursing Studies*, 47(6), 761-769.

Wilson, R. D., & Australian Human Rights and Equal Opportunity Commission. (1997). *Bringing them home: National Inquiry into the Separation of Aboriginal and Torres Strait Islander Children from their Families.* Sydney: Human Rights and Equal Opportunity Commission.

Zalta, E. N. (Ed.). (2008). *The Stanford encyclopedia of philosophy.* Stanford: Center for the Study of Language and Information, Stanford University. https://plato.stanford.edu/cite.html

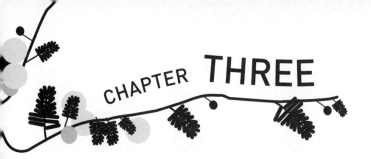

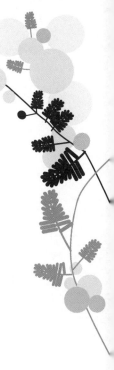

CHAPTER THREE

Frameworks of healthcare

Michael Curtin, Caroline Robinson and Norman Dulvarie

LEARNING CONCEPTS

Studying this chapter should enable you to:

1. identify differences between Western and Aboriginal and Torres Strait Islander peoples' concepts of health and social and emotional wellbeing.
2. explain the biomedical, biopsychosocial, ICF and socio-ecological frameworks of health and wellbeing.
3. discuss the conflict of applying Western frameworks of health and wellbeing to health service delivery for Aboriginal and Torres Strait Islander peoples.
4. evaluate the interdependent connections between the seven domains comprising the model of social and emotional wellbeing for Aboriginal and Torres Strait Islander peoples.
5. discuss the factors that inform effective provision of health and wellbeing services to Aboriginal and Torres Strait Islander peoples.

KEY TERMS

Aboriginal Community Controlled Health Service (ACCHS)

Indigenous health

Indigenous concept of social and emotional wellbeing

Introduction

The intention of the Australian healthcare system is to provide universal and accessible care. Health services are provided in a variety of locations, including hospitals and health centres, and are delivered by a range of public, private and not-for-profit providers that are funded by federal, state and local government (Isbel & Jamieson, 2017). The initial point of contact for people to the healthcare system is most often through the primary healthcare (PHC) sector. General practitioners (GPs) provide a range of primary healthcare services and are the gatekeepers for secondary healthcare, which is provided by hospitals, rehabilitation centres, specialists and community-based services (Fisher, Baum, Kay & Frie, 2017).

The range of health services and the accessibility of healthcare can differ significantly based on where people live, the availability of health professionals, and the pressure that hospitals and other health services are under (Isbel & Jamieson, 2017). Despite the intent to provide appropriate and acceptable health services that are physically and economically accessible, healthcare can be inaccessible for some people in Australia (Ware, 2013). Clients may be unaware of available services, and physical and economic barriers may further impede their access to appropriate healthcare. In addition, health services can be inaccessible to clients if providers do not acknowledge and respect different perspectives, particularly non-Western views of health and wellbeing. This can result in inappropriate, unacceptable and inaccessible healthcare services for Aboriginal and Torres Strait Islander peoples.

In a review of primary healthcare from the perspective of Aboriginal and Torres Strait Islander peoples, Gomersall et al. (2017) found that the 'inadequate access to primary healthcare services responsive to Indigenous clients' holistic needs, modifiable socio-economic factors, including low income, poor education, poor living conditions and social exclusion, are principal contributors to the higher chronic disease burden in the Indigenous population' (p. 417). Health and social inequity for Aboriginal and Torres Strait Islander peoples means that they experience a burden of disease two and a half times greater than non-Indigenous Australian people (Thompson, Talley & Kong, 2017; Wilson, Kelly, Magarey, Jones & Mackean, 2016). The comparably poorer health status and shorter life expectancy of Aboriginal and Torres Strait Islander peoples is a consequence of the long-term, intergenerational impact of colonisation and the brutal, racist and discriminatory past (and current) policies of governments (Bailie et al., 2017; Blignault & Williams, 2017; Wilson et al., 2016). Colonisation led to the removal of Aboriginal and Torres Strait Islander peoples from their countries, spiritually, socially and economically alienating them from their lands, their communities, and the general population (Duckett, 2007; Gilroy, Dew, Lincoln & Hines, 2017):

> The process of colonisation traumatically disrupted sources of social and emotional wellbeing within cultures, communities, and families, with resulting intergenerational mental health impacts. All these effects are exacerbated by the

negative impact of social determinants today. Colonisation and the disruption of cultural, family, and community life through dispossession and other often violent acts such as the forced removal of children from families (the Stolen Generations) have affected generations of Aboriginal and Torres Strait Islander people and intergenerational trauma has emerged as a significant issue requiring attention.

Calma, Dudgeon and Bray (2017, p. 255)

The intergenerational impact of colonisation on the social and emotional wellbeing of Aboriginal and Torres Strait Islander peoples is a key reason why their healthcare and support needs differ significantly from those of non-Indigenous Australian people (Lindeman, Mackell, Lin, Farthing, Jensen, Meredith & Haralambous, 2017). Furthermore, healthcare services based on Western frameworks of health do not align with Aboriginal and Torres Strait Islander peoples' beliefs about health and wellbeing. Inevitably, these types of health services do not address the health needs of Aboriginal and Torres Strait Islander peoples (Duckett, 2007; McCalman, Bainbridge, Percival & Tsey, 2016).

Aboriginal and Torres Strait Islander peoples' perceptions of health

Indigenous constructs of health pre-date Western beliefs about health and illness by tens of thousands of years (Gormon, Nielsen & Best, 2006). Indigenous perspectives of health 'are based on cultural values, beliefs and traditions passed down over generations, [and involve believing that] holism is core to understanding health and well-being [empathising] the interconnected nature of all life, the environment and the cosmos' (Priest, Thompson, Mackean, Baker & Waters, 2017, p. 632). This is in stark contrast to the mainstream Western health and medical contexts that mainly centre on 'bio-reductionist empirical' frameworks (Priest et al., 2017, p. 632). A Western model of health that privileges physical and psychological elements, but does not acknowledge spirituality, culture and connection to the environment, will fail Aboriginal and Torres Strait Islander peoples (Priest et al., 2017). Blignault and Williams (2017) and the National Aboriginal Health Strategy Working Party (1989) state that an Aboriginal and Torres Strait Islander peoples' definition of health embraces factors that impact on the health and wellbeing of individuals, communities and broader society. These factors include culture, justice, safety, employment and arts, and have a strong basis in the connections between people and their families, communities and history. Acknowledging the broad cultural diversity among Aboriginal and Torres Strait Islander peoples, traditional health beliefs are grounded in the interconnectedness of multiple aspects of life, including kinship relationships and religion. There is an emphasis on social and spiritual dysfunction as a cause of illness.

Indigenous health
'Not just the physical wellbeing of the individual but the social, emotional and cultural wellbeing of the whole community in which each individual is able to achieve their full potential as a human being, thereby bringing about the total wellbeing of their Community' (National Aboriginal Health and Strategy Working Party, 1989, p. x).

The definition of **Indigenous health** generally accepted by Aboriginal and Torres Strait Islander peoples is the one proposed by the National Aboriginal Health and Strategy Working Party (1989, p. x):

> Not just the physical wellbeing of the individual but the social, emotional and cultural wellbeing of the whole community in which each individual is able to achieve their full potential as a human being, thereby bringing about the total wellbeing of their Community. This is a whole-of-life view and it also includes the cyclical concept of life-death-life.

When referring to health, Aboriginal and Torres Strait Islander peoples refer to social and emotional wellbeing (Jackson King & Dender, 2017). The World Health Organization (2011) defines social and emotional wellbeing as a state of wellbeing perceived by the person based on the person's awareness of his/her ability to cope with health issues, and their being able to productively work and contribute to his/her community. However, Aboriginal and Torres Strait Islander peoples find this definition to be limited and too person-focused (Casey, 2014). Gomersall et al. (2017) suggest that from the perspectives of Aboriginal and Torres Strait Islander peoples, health is conceived in a holistic way that 'incorporates body, mind, spirit, land, environment, custom, socio-economic status, family and community' (p. 417). Hence, Aboriginal and Torres Strait Islander peoples see social and emotional wellbeing as reflective of their holistic view of health and see the impact that a wide range of experiences and life events can have on their health (Calma et al., 2017; Le Grande, Ski, Thompson, Scuffham, Kularatna, Jackson & Brown, 2017). Social and emotional wellbeing is a dynamic concept as it changes throughout a person's life and will be interpreted differently by individuals, communities and different cultural groups (Gee, Dudgeon, Schultz, Hart & Kelly, 2014). What is common to this concept is the acknowledgment that a positive sense of social and emotional wellbeing is essential for Aboriginal and Torres Strait Islander peoples to lead successful and fulfilling lives (Commonwealth of Australia, 2017).

Indigenous concept of social and emotional wellbeing Connects the health of Aboriginal and Torres Strait Islander peoples to the health of their family, kin and community, and their connection to country, culture, spirituality and ancestry (Calma, Dudgeon & Bray, 2017).

Calma et al. (2017, p. 256) state that the **Indigenous concept of social and emotional wellbeing**:

> connects the health of Aboriginal and Torres Strait Islander individuals to the health of their family, kin, community, and their connection to country, culture, spirituality, and ancestry. Social and emotional wellbeing is a deep-rooted, more collective and holistic concept of health and mental health than Western concepts. The Aboriginal and Torres Strait Islander social and emotional wellbeing concept also accommodates experiential differences: the disproportionate impact of poor physical health, lower income, unemployment, racism, lower educational attainment, poor and overcrowded housing and other social and cultural determinants on Aboriginal and Torres Strait Islander individuals, families, and communities when compared to the non-Indigenous population.

In Australia today, the funding and delivery of healthcare is founded primarily on Western frameworks of health. It is important to critically evaluate these frameworks of health in order to understand the differing expectations of health service delivery and healthcare between Aboriginal and Torres Strait Islander peoples and non-Indigenous Australians.

Western frameworks of health

Health is a dynamic and elusive concept (Taylor, 2008a) as there are 'unique individual, family, social and cultural contexts in which the term is used' (Liamputtong, Fanany & Verrinder, 2012, p. 2). The Australian Institute of Health and Welfare (2014) states: 'Health, or being in good health, is important to everyone [influencing] not just how we feel, but how we function and participate in the community' (p. 3). This definition signifies health as a basic human right for all people regardless of race, religion or political beliefs, as stated in the 1948 United Nations Universal Declaration of Human Rights (Taylor, 2008a).

Rather than confining 'health' to a simple definition, Taylor (2008b) proposed four frameworks to conceptualise health and wellbeing:

1 biomedical
2 biopsychosocial
3 International Classification of Functioning, Disability and Health (ICF)
4 socio-ecological.

These health frameworks are 'underpinned by differing conceptualisations of core constructs like health, illness and wellbeing, which become translated into health policy, service delivery and professional practice' (Taylor, 2008b, pp. 23–24). A summary of each of these frameworks follows.

Biomedical framework of health

The biomedical framework of health emerged in the eighteenth and nineteenth centuries in line with the move towards rational and logical thinking, away from knowledge based on religious scripture (Wilcock & Hocking, 2015). This framework underpinned the development and provision of traditional Western health services and is based on the premise that there are two states of being: a healthy state, in which there is no illness; and an ill state, in which there is the presence of illness (Germov, 2018; Taylor, 2008b). The focus of treatment is on fixing the malfunction of one of the body's biological systems that is diagnosed to have caused the illness (Germov, 2018). The adoption of this framework led to health services becoming more mechanistic as assessments and interventions were focused on body structures and functions, treating the illness, and using quantitative measures for monitoring improvement (Gillen & Greber, 2014; Hocking, 2013).

The biopsychosocial and ICF frameworks of health

The World Health Organization describes health as 'a state of complete physical, mental and social wellbeing and not merely the absence of disease or infirmity' (1948, p. 1). The important aspect of this definition is that it marks a significant shift from health being the absence of illness (the focus of the biomedical model) to health being each person's subjective perception of, and satisfaction with, their life—whether or not they have an illness (King, 2014). It is this understanding of health that led to the development of the biopsychosocial view of health (Germov, 2018), and laid the foundations for the development of health promotion as a health intervention strategy, and strategies for the prevention of illness (Wilcock & Hocking, 2015).

The biopsychosocial framework is different from the biomedical framework as it is underpinned by system theory: it is a multi-factorial model of illness that takes into account biological, psychological and social factors (Germov, 2018). It is based on the premise that health is determined by the dynamic interaction of a person's body structures and functions, subjective behaviours, beliefs, thought processes, motivations and experiences, and culture, family, community and society (Germov, 2018). This framework led to the development of the International Classification of Impairments, Disabilities and Handicaps (ICIDH) by the World Health Organization in 1980 (Peterson, Mpofu & Oakland, 2010) and the categorisation of the consequences of disease according to three dimensions: structural and functional body impairments, disabilities, and handicaps. Impairment was defined as a problem with a person's body function and structure, disability as a result of the affected body function and structure, and handicap as the limitations experienced in the environment because of the affected body function and structure. Although some consideration was given to the impact of social and psychological factors, this framework focused on treatments to make a person's body structure and function as 'normal' as possible. A positive outcome of the adoption of the biopsychosocial framework was the introduction of the concept of 'wellbeing': 'a broader concept than health as it typically involve[d] a person's sense of overall satisfaction with ... life' (Taylor, 2008a, pp. 11–12). This meant that a person's health status included subjective experiences of quality of life (King, 2014), in that a person may have an illness and feel healthy, or a person may not have an illness and feel unhealthy (Liamputtong et al., 2012).

Although the biopsychosocial framework of health was an advance on the biomedical framework, it was replaced by the International Classification of Functioning, Disability and Health (ICF), a framework that proposed health existed along a continuum rather than being a static state fixed in time, and was a result of dynamic interactions between the person and the person's environment (Alford, Remedios, Webb & Ewen, 2013; Taylor, 2008b). Although the ICF was still individually focused, it acknowledged the impact of internal and external factors on an individual's health (Alford et al., 2013;

Peterson et al., 2010). According to the ICF, impairment results from changes to a person's body functions and structures, and leads to activity limitations (that is, a person experiencing difficulty executing a task or action) and participation restrictions (that is, the difficulty a person has doing things such as work, recreational and leisure activities, and personal care). A graphic illustration of the ICF is depicted in Figure 3.1 and a brief description of the components of the ICF can be found in Table 3.1.

Figure 3.1 International Classification of Functioning, Disability and Health (ICF)

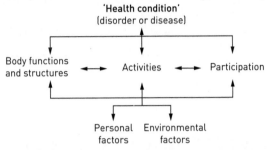

Source: World Health Organization (2001).

Table 3.1 Description of components of the ICF

ICF components	Description of component
Health condition	This refers to a person's diagnosed disorder and/or disease. The World Health Organization defines health as 'the complete physical, mental and social functioning of a person and not merely the absence of disease' (World Health Organization, 1948, Preamble).
Functioning	Functioning refers to the 'dynamic interaction between a person's health condition, environment factors and personal factors' (World Health Organization, 2013, p. 5). When a person's functioning is affected this is referred to as a 'disability'. This term encompasses impairments, limitations to activities and/or restrictions to participation (Petersen, Mpofu & Oakland, 2010; World Health Organization, 2001).
Body functions and structures	Body functions refers to the physiological, neurological and psychological systems that enable the body to work. Body structures refers to the anatomical parts of the body. When a person's body functions or body structures are affected this is referred to as an 'impairment'.
Activity	Activity refers to the doing of a task or an action by a person. When a person has difficulty in the doing of a task or an action, this is referred to as an 'activity limitation'.
Participation	Participation refers to the involvement of a person in various occupations and life roles. When a person has difficulty or is unable to be involved in occupations and life roles, this is referred to as a 'participation restriction'.

(Continued)

ICF components	Description of component
Personal factors	The ICF does not provide a clear definition of personal factors because of the complex nature of social and cultural variation (Peterson, Mpofu & Oakland, 2010). It is suggested that personal factors could include such things as ethnicity, gender, age, educational level, psychological assets, habits, social background and lifestyle (Wilcock & Hocking, 2015).
Environmental factors	These factors refer to the physical (natural and manufactured), social (relationships with family, friends and communities) and attitudinal (policies, services, rules and laws) environments in which people live. Environmental factors can either facilitate or inhibit an individual's functioning.

Based on definitions provided by the World Health Organization (2001).

Socio-ecological framework of health

According to Taylor (2008b), the socio-ecological framework maximises 'health at all levels within society, from the individual to the whole community [and promotes] health rather than simply responding to illness after it has developed' (p. 41). This framework differs from the previous frameworks because it focuses on the prevention and social responsibility of illness, and the promotion of health and wellbeing, moving beyond the medical treatment of an individual and of medical conditions. While the need for medical treatment for biological and physiological aspects of illness is recognised, it is acknowledged that this should occur within a social context.

Another term used for this framework is 'public health', as the focus is on determinants of health and the implementation of interventions at group, community, population and organisation levels (Germov, 2018; Taylor, 2008b). Public health strategies are based on social justice principles (Hume Chambers & Walker, 2012) and focus on the health of groups, communities, populations and organisations, taking into account the interaction between the multiple social determinants of health (Moll, Gewurtz, Krupa & Law, 2013). This is in keeping with the right people have to a high standard of health and healthcare (Taket, 2012; United Nations, 1948) that is not dependent on their ethnicity, religious or political beliefs, and/or economic or social condition (Wilcock & Hocking, 2015).

The move to improve the health of populations and the focus on health promotion strategies is an outcome of the World Health Organization's (1978) *Primary Health Care* report of the International Conference at Alma Alta, and is underpinned by the World Health Organization's *Ottawa Charter of Health Promotion* (World Health Organization, Health and Welfare Canada & Canadian Public Health Association, 1986), a charter aimed at promoting good health of groups, communities, populations and organisations. This charter is underpinned by an understanding of the social determinants of health (Jirojwong & Liamputtong, 2009a, 2009b), which the World Health Organization (2013) considers to be the main cause of health status inequalities seen among groups of people living within a country and also between countries.

The Australian Institute of Health and Welfare (2014) uses a diagram to illustrate the social, economic, political, cultural and environmental factors that impact on and determine health (see Figure 3.2). Within this figure it can be seen that the determinants are separated into four groups impacting a person's health and wellbeing over time, with the direction of determinants moving from left to right. The determinants are associated with factors that facilitate good health or lead to poor health (Rumbold & Dickson-Swift, 2012; Taylor, 2008b).

Figure 3.2 A framework for the determinants of health

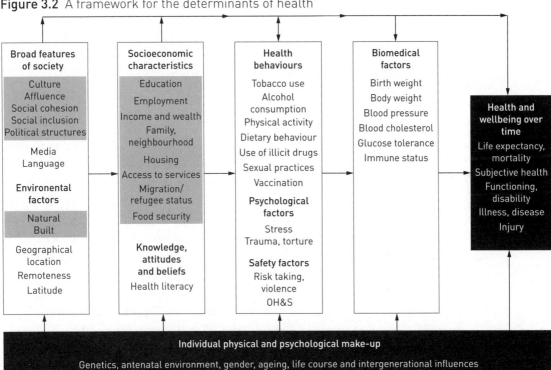

Note: Grey shading highlights selected social determinants of health

Source: Australian Institute of Health and Welfare (2014). Reproduced with permission.

One of the outcomes of the focus on population health has been a growing understanding of the cultural influence on health. A focus on population health, health equality and determinants of health highlights the disparity between the health of people from different cultures, and also the inappropriateness of imposing Western frameworks of health (that is, the biomedical, biopsychosocial and ICF frameworks) on people from non-Western backgrounds.

The biomedical, biopsychosocial and ICF frameworks and the health of Aboriginal and Torres Strait Islander peoples

Australian healthcare services are predominantly based on the biomedical, biopyschosocial and ICF frameworks of health. These frameworks have been criticised for not being relevant to Aboriginal and Torres Strait Islander peoples, as these frameworks do not align to their view of health. The reductionist nature of the biomedical framework means that it does not provide a sound 'explanation of who becomes ill and who stays healthy, as it does not account for the complex interplay of personal, environmental, psychological, physiological and occupational factors that impact on health' (Wilcock & Hocking, 2015, p. 67). It contributes to numerous negative outcomes, such as the objectification of people who are referred to by the name of the health condition they have or as 'patient', becoming passive recipients of 'expert' advice and treatment. It does not take into account the impact of history, colonisation, disconnection from land, community, and the subjective and collective view of health and wellbeing.

Criticisms of the biopsychosocial and the ICF frameworks revolve around the focus on the individual and the categorisation of people based on assumptions of there being a 'normal' state (Conti-Becker, 2009; Hemmingsson & Jonsson, 2005; Whalley Hammell, 2004). This focus on 'normality' creates hierarchical experts who make judgments on what can be considered normal and what is deviant, leading to exclusion, marginalisation and stigmatisation. In addition, there is little consideration of the impact of environmental factors such as poverty, inadequate or absent services, abuse and neglect in all its forms, and other very common social and economic problems (Bickehbach, 2014). The inability to acknowledge the impact of these environmental factors means that a full understanding of the multiple determinants of health is not evident, with the biopsychosocial framework and the ICF predominantly focusing on the individual rather than on the social factors that impact on the health of groups and populations. This is particularly relevant as one claim of the biopsychosocial and the ICF frameworks is that they could be used for all people and they are applicable to all cultures (Australian Institute of Health and Welfare, 2014; World Health Organization, 2001). Gilroy, Donelly, Colmar and Parmenter (2013) contest this assertion stating that these frameworks do not pay 'enough attention to how the experience of colonisation influences the way that [health and] disability is conceptualised, understood and experienced in Indigenous communities' (p. 43). Hence, the biopsychosocial and ICF frameworks do not capture and include Aboriginal and Torres Strait Islander peoples' perceptions and experiences of health and social and emotional wellbeing; rather, Western health labels and categorisations are imposed on all cultures and societies.

Aboriginal and Torres Strait Islander peoples' cultural ways of knowing and understanding health and social and emotional wellbeing identifies an ideological conflict with Western biomedical, biopsychosocial and ICF frameworks of health (Foster, 2008; Le Grande et al., 2017). Through the process of colonisation, these Western frameworks of health have been imposed on Aboriginal and Torres Strait Islander peoples, causing significant conflict with their traditional practices that reinforced the intimate connection between mind, body, spirit and cosmos. The continuing strong influence of the biomedical, biopsychosocial and ICF frameworks on Western health practice, and the reliance on evidence-based principles with knowledge organised according to different health disciplines, is at odds with the holistic approach to health and wellbeing practiced by many non-Western people (Kendall, Milliken, Barnet & Marshall, 2008). Western frameworks of health promote racism and stigmatisation as they do not account for the dignity, self-esteem and self-determination of Aboriginal and Torres Strait Islander peoples' cultures and ways of knowing (Ward & Gorman, 2010). This in turn negatively impacts on Aboriginal and Torres Strait Islander peoples' social and emotional wellbeing (Le Grande et al., 2017).

The socio-ecological framework and the health of Aboriginal and Torres Strait Islander peoples

Of the four Western health frameworks described by Taylor (2008b), only the socio-ecological framework of health encourages health professionals to look beyond working with individuals who have an illness and embrace population health and wellness (Wilcock & Hocking, 2015). This framework encourages health services and professionals to develop a stronger social justice approach to practice and to acknowledge that health and wellbeing are influenced by factors that operate at the individual, interpersonal, community and societal levels. Whalley Hammell and Iwama (2012) argue that the focus on health and wellbeing in this framework resonates with people from different cultures, as the concept of wellbeing, although interpreted differently, can align with the perceptions of health held by people from non-Western cultural backgrounds. This is the case for Aboriginal and Torres Strait Islander peoples, who view the concept of social and emotional wellbeing as synonymous with the term 'health' (Blignault & Williams, 2017; Gee, Dudgeon, Schultz, Hart & Kelly, 2014).

The concept of social and emotional wellbeing

A model of social and emotional wellbeing relevant to Aboriginal and Torres Strait Islander peoples has been proposed by Gee et al. (2014) (see Figure 3.3). In proposing this model, the authors state that social and emotional wellbeing is a multi-faceted concept based on a holistic view of health. The authors argue that for Aboriginal

Figure 3.3 Social and emotional wellbeing from the perspective of Aboriginal and Torres Strait Islander peoples

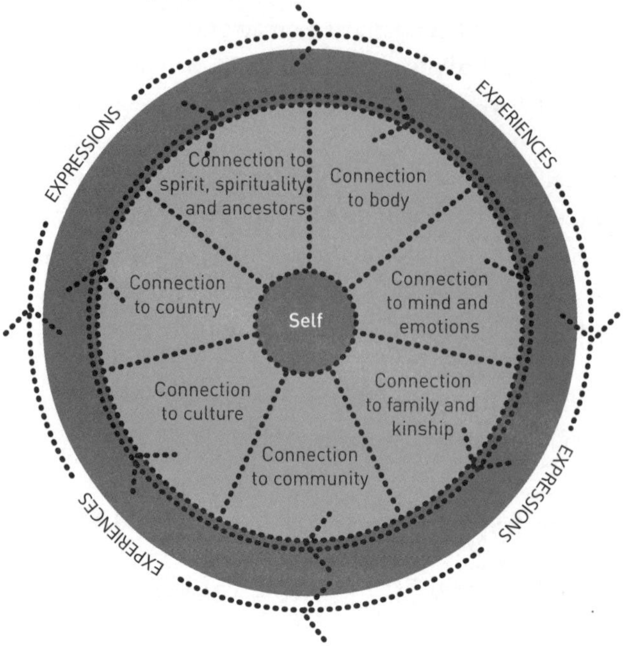

Source: Gee et al. (2014, p. 57). Reproduced with permission.

and Torres Strait Islander peoples, social and emotional wellbeing is intricately and intrinsically linked to the interdependent connections each person has to seven domains (body; mind and emotions; family and kinship; community; culture; country; and spirit, spirituality and ancestors), how these connections have been shaped across generations, and the processes by which they affect the individual. Gee et al. (2014) proposed the phrase 'social and emotional wellbeing' as it more meaningfully represents 'health' for Aboriginal and Torres Strait Islander peoples, signifying 'a relatively distinct set of wellbeing domains and principles, and an increasingly documented set of culturally informed practices that differ in important ways with how the term is understood and used within Western health discourse' (pp. 56–57). This model of social and emotional wellbeing is informed by nine guiding principles presented in the *Social and Emotional Well Being Framework* document (Social Health Reference Group, 2004). These principles shape Aboriginal and Torres Strait Islander peoples' conceptualisations of social and emotional wellbeing and identify core cultural values (see Table 3.2).

Gee et al. (2014) state that a person's social and emotional wellbeing is influenced not just by their connections to each of the seven domains in the model but also by historical and socio-political determinants that have underpinned the intergenerational trauma experienced by Aboriginal and Torres Strait Islander peoples. These historical and socio-political determinants include 'environmental deprivation; emotional,

Table 3.2 Social and emotional wellbeing framework: nine guiding principles

1.	Health as holistic
2.	The right to self-determination
3.	The need for cultural understanding
4.	The impact of history in trauma and loss
5.	Recognition of human rights
6.	The impact of racism and stigma
7.	Recognition of the centrality of kinship
8.	Recognition of cultural diversity
9.	Recognition of Aboriginal strengths

NB: Readers are advised to refer to the Social Health Reference Group (2004) for further explanation of these principles.

Source: Calma et al. (2017).

physical and sexual abuse; emotional and physical neglect; stress; social exclusion; grief and trauma; removal from family; substance abuse; family breakdowns; cultural disconnection; racism; discrimination; domestic violence; and social disadvantage' (Day & Francisco, 2013, p. 350). Disruption of these connections, particularly as a result of historical and political impacts of colonisation, have negatively impacted the social and emotional wellbeing of individuals, families and communities (Gee et al., 2014), as evidenced by social determinants such as low socio-economic status, poverty, poor education achievement and unemployment among Aboriginal and Torres Strait Islander peoples and communities.

To positively impact on the social and emotional wellbeing of Aboriginal and Torres Strait Islander peoples, health services need to respect cultural ways of knowing, being and doing, and support the dignity, self-esteem and self-determination of Aboriginal and Torres Strait Islander peoples and communities, giving them control over the health services (Gormon et al., 2006). Davy, Kite, Aitken, Dodd, Rigney, Hayes and Van Emden (2016) suggest that the social and emotional wellbeing of Aboriginal and Torres Strait Islander peoples can be supported by providing health services that maintain Indigenous identity, promote independence and deliver culturally safe care. Aboriginal and Torres Strait Islander peoples who are able to maintain their connections to family, community and country are generally more likely to maintain a strong inner spirit (Casey, 2014). A strong inner spirit ensures social and emotional wellbeing and positive decision making, impacting not only on the individual but also making the whole community strong (Casey, 2014). This has particular resonance when deciding the extent to which self-determination or assimilation should inform the guiding principles for policies related to the health of Aboriginal and Torres Strait Islander peoples (Foster & Fleming, 2008).

What works in Aboriginal and Torres Strait Islander peoples' health?

In order for health services to meet the needs of Aboriginal and Torres Strait Islander peoples, it is important that there is community ownership and control; clinical and managerial input from Aboriginal and Torres Strait Islander staff; and delivery of models of care that embrace Indigenous knowledge systems (Gomersall et al., 2017). To be effective in reducing the burden of chronic illness and improving health outcomes for Aboriginal and Torres Strait Islander peoples, health professionals and health services must consider 'community, economic and social development, self-reliance and self-determination, [with] the provision of basic needs extending beyond clinical health services' (Schultz & Cairney, 2017, p. 2). Wakerman and Shannon (2016) propose multiple strategies for ensuring that health services meet the needs of Aboriginal and Torres Strait Islander peoples, which include the provision of service models that are funded adequately and that focus on Indigenous knowledge systems and socio-cultural needs. It is important to focus on the prevention of ill-health and the development of a 'whole-of-system approach and policy consistency' (Wakerman & Shannon, 2016, p. 364), in order to create stable health systems and better coordinated services and programs (Thomas, Williams, Ritchie & Zwi, 2015) that emphasise the strength and resilience of Aboriginal and Torres Strait Islander peoples and foster self-determination (Jackson King & Dender, 2017).

Effective health services embrace the social and emotional wellbeing model (see Figure 3.3) (Gee et al., 2014) and the nine guiding principles of the social and emotional wellbeing framework (see Table 3.2) (Calma et al., 2017). The principles inherent in this model and framework embody a whole-of-life view of health held by Aboriginal and Torres Strait Islander peoples. Health and wellbeing programs developed or implemented in accordance with the nine guiding principles are 'more likely to be effective and have positive outcomes than those that do not', as they promote 'self-determination and community governance, reconnection and community life, restoration and community resilience' (Dudgeon, Purdie, Walker & Calma, 2014, p. 2). Healthcare is effective when 'multi-dimensional solutions are provided, which build on existing community, family and individual strengths and capacity and may include counselling and social support, culturally informed practice and, where necessary, support during family reunification' (Commonwealth of Australia, 2017, p. 7).

Aboriginal Community Controlled Health Services (ACCHSs) offer an effective model of health service delivery in Australia, as they are developed on the principles of community ownership and control, employ clinical and managerial Aboriginal and Torres Strait Islander staff, and implement models of care that embrace Aboriginal and Torres Strait Islander peoples' knowledge systems. ACCHSs empower Aboriginal and Torres Strait Islander peoples by enabling community control over the health services they receive, which affords the opportunity to address institutional racism,

Aboriginal Community Controlled Health Service (ACCHS) A primary healthcare service operated by an Aboriginal community to deliver culturally appropriate healthcare to the community that controls it.

marginalisation and inequitable access to mainstream health services (Tsey, Whiteside, Haswell-Elkins, Bainbridge, Cadet-James & Wilson, 2010). A brief overview of ACCHSs is provided in Case study 3.1.

Offering culturally safe mainstream health services to Aboriginal and Torres Strait Islander peoples

Not all Aboriginal and Torres Strait Islander people can access an ACCHS, and not all available health services can be offered through an ACCHS, so it is important that non-Indigenous health services apply principles that ensure delivery of culturally safe and relevant services to Aboriginal and Torres Strait Islander peoples.

All health professionals have a role to play in reducing the health disparities between Aboriginal and Torres Strait Islander peoples and non-Indigenous Australians. Through a lack of understanding and acceptance of Aboriginal and Torres Strait Islander peoples' knowledge and ways of doing and being, the attitudes and approach of many non-Indigenous health professionals perpetuates institutional racism and the continuing poor health of Aboriginal and Torres Strait Islander peoples (Hill, Ewen, Paul & Wilkin, 2017). From an Aboriginal and Torres Strait Islander peoples' perspective, health services based on Western frameworks continue to create barriers to appropriate healthcare and negatively impact social and emotional wellbeing. Western frameworks of health make it more difficult for Aboriginal and Torres Strait Islander peoples to access, afford and navigate healthcare services and systems (Davy et al., 2016). It is essential for health professionals to understand health and wellbeing from Aboriginal and Torres Strait Islander peoples' perspectives, in order to remove barriers and facilitate access to healthcare services and systems (Davy et al., 2016): 'Improving health professionals' understandings of Indigenous peoples' cultures and the factors that support their health and well-being is likely to improve not only the acceptability of primary healthcare and aged-care services but also the quality of care they provide' (p. 90). All health professionals who work with Aboriginal and Torres Strait Islander peoples must work towards improving accessibility and quality of care for their clients (Gomersall et al., 2017) and understand the 'importance of a holistic approach to health care that takes into account the social, emotional, cultural and economic contexts of people's lives' (Francis-Cracknell, Gilby & Adams, 2017, p. 46). This means that non-Indigenous Australian health workers should move initially towards adopting the socio-ecological framework of health to underpin their practice, and embrace the social and emotional wellbeing concepts of health relevant to Aboriginal and Torres Strait Islander peoples and the nine guiding principles in the *Social and Emotional Well Being Framework* document (Social Health Reference Group, 2004; see Table 3.2).

By embracing these principles, health professionals will be able to support Aboriginal and Torres Strait Islander peoples to retain and regain control:

> [W]hich includes the ability to maintain identity and culture, to base community structures on custom and traditional law, and to have the capacity for local decision making and implementation. Effective engagement then facilitates external assistance to contribute to the future aspirations of Aboriginal and Torres Strait Islander peoples, rather than to define the processes of how Aboriginal and Torres Strait Islander peoples are included.
>
> Thorpe, Arabena, Sullivan, Silburn and Rowley (2016, p. 1)

IMPLICATIONS FOR NURSING AND ALLIED HEALTH PRACTICE

- Western frameworks of health are not relevant to Aboriginal and Torres Strait Islander peoples as these frameworks do not align with their perspectives of health and social and emotional wellbeing.
- Embrace Aboriginal and Torres Strait Islander peoples' understanding of health and social and emotional wellbeing and the nine guiding principles of the social and emotional wellbeing framework.
- Engage with Aboriginal and Torres Strait Islander peoples to foster self-determination and the provision of culturally safe health services.
- Best practice requires working collaboratively, and in partnership, with ACCHSs in the provision of healthcare for Aboriginal and Torres Strait Islander peoples.
- Non-Indigenous health practitioners must engage in personal and professional development to inform culturally safe best practice when working with Aboriginal and Torres Strait Islander peoples.

Case study 3.1

Overview of Aboriginal Community Controlled Health Services (ACCHSs)

Aboriginal Community Controlled Health Services (ACCHSs) were established because mainstream health services and systems based on Western health frameworks could not provide appropriate healthcare for Aboriginal and Torres Strait Islander peoples. Aboriginal and Torres Strait Islander peoples have indicated that their Indigenous identity is challenged and denied when accessing mainstream health services; they have felt discriminated against, patronised, assaulted and threatened.

The first Aboriginal Medical Service (AMS) was initiated on a voluntary basis in Redfern, Sydney in 1971. There are now 143 ACCHSs across Australia and these are represented by a peak body, the National Aboriginal Community Controlled Health Organisation (NACCHO). All these ACCHSs contribute to more positive health outcomes for Aboriginal and Torres Strait Islander peoples compared with mainstream health services as they provide culturally and clinically safe primary healthcare to Aboriginal and Torres Strait Islander peoples and communities (Ah Chee, Boffa & Tilton, 2016; Dwyer, O'Donnell, Willis & Kelly, 2016). ACCHSs provide culturally appropriate, comprehensive primary healthcare empowering Aboriginal and Torres Strait Islander peoples and communities to increase self-efficacy and improve their health (McFarlane, Devine, Judd, Nichols & Watt, 2017).

ACCHSs have been identified as ideal models of comprehensive primary healthcare as they integrate clinical care, health promotion and community capacity building in culturally safe and respectful ways (Caffery, Bradford, Wickramasinghe, Hayman & Smith, 2017). Wakerman and Shannon (2016) suggest that ACCHSs have developed a model of primary healthcare 'that seeks to focus on prevention and health promotion … to address the social determinants of health. There is evidence that such models positively influence access and other outcomes. This has undoubtedly been a positive response to health and social needs' (p. 363).

Gomersall et al. (2017) stated that ACCHSs have been found to be effective in improving health outcomes for Aboriginal and Torres Strait Islander peoples and communities because these services:

1. are accessible in terms of being a welcoming and culturally safe space
2. deliver healthcare in a culturally safe and respectful way
3. are comprehensive and tailored to meet the holistic needs of Aboriginal and Torres Strait Islander peoples and communities.

In addition, ACCHSs are effective because they are incorporated and governed by an elected Aboriginal body, employ an Aboriginal managerial and clinical workforce where possible, and deliver holistic and culturally appropriate health services that embrace Aboriginal and Torres Strait Islander peoples' knowledge systems (Gomersall et al., 2017; Stewart, Sanson-Fisher, Eades & Fitzgerald, 2012; Tsey et al., 2010). ACCHSs are independent from government and 'represent self-determination in the provision of comprehensive primary health care to Aboriginal and Torres Strait Islander people' (Stewart et al., 2012, p. 618). This community control of resources and decision making is considered essential to improving Aboriginal and Torres Strait Islander peoples' health outcomes as it empowers Aboriginal and Torres Strait Islander

(Continued)

OXFORD UNIVERSITY PRESS

individuals, families and communities, strengthens connection to culture, and reduces damaging effects of colonisation and government policies (Blignault & Williams, 2017; Tsey et al., 2010).

Further information about ACCHSs can be found at the National Aboriginal Community Controlled Health Organisation website: https://www.naccho. org.au.

CRITICAL REFLECTION QUESTIONS

- What do you understand by the term 'institutionalised racism' in relation to health service delivery?
- How does the integrated primary healthcare model adopted by ACCHSs align with the model of social and emotional wellbeing (Gee et al., 2014)?
- What is the location of the ACCHS closest to where you live or work and what range of health services is provided?

Case study 3.2

Albury Wodonga Aboriginal Health Service

The Albury Wodonga Aboriginal Health Service (AWAHS) outreach service operates from a van in the rural city of Wangaratta, in northeast Victoria. For one day each week, a non-Indigenous doctor and an Aboriginal Health Practitioner (AHP) assess local Aboriginal clients in the well-equipped van. In addition to providing a health service, the AHP also has an important role as a cultural broker for the Aboriginal clients. Consistency is key to the success of this outreach service—it takes place in the same place, at the same time, with the same staff each week.

All treatments provided through this service are bulk-billed and a client may be referred back to AWAHS for follow-up. Importantly, there are no out-of-pocket expenses for a client. This is a critical factor to encourage potential clients to engage with the service. Client numbers continue to grow each week, with a current maximum of 11 clients engaging with the service each day. Importantly, the 30-minute appointment times provide plenty of time for each client to tell their story.

Clients tell stories of their experiences of institutionalised racism and judgmental staff in mainstream health services. They talk about the conscious and unconscious bias displayed by non-Indigenous health professionals when they identify as an Aboriginal person. Their stories indicate that if no effort is made by a health service to be culturally safe, clients will not identify as an Aboriginal person and this can be a hindrance to their healthcare.

This outreach initiative has demonstrated a need for this service in the Wangaratta Aboriginal community. The target is for the AWAHS outreach service to become self-sufficient through Medicare funding. This could lead to the inception of a permanent Aboriginal Medical Service (AMS) in Wangaratta. However, the challenge is to remain true to the principles of primary healthcare as the risk is that a Medicare-driven model for Aboriginal and Torres Strait Islander peoples' healthcare could compromise the service; for example, through reduced appointment times.

A range of stakeholders has enabled the realisation of this outreach service. Stakeholders including the Poche Centre for Indigenous Health at the University of Sydney, AWAHS and the Rural Workforce Agency Victoria have provided funding towards the cost of the van, and the salaries of the doctor and the AHP.

CRITICAL REFLECTION QUESTIONS

- What is unconscious bias? How may this bias influence your practice as a health professional?
- What Aboriginal health services are available in the area in which you live and work? What is the scope of practice of an Aboriginal Health Practitioner as compared to an Aboriginal Health Worker?
- From a social justice perspective, how could you contribute locally to make a difference for Aboriginal and Torres Strait Islander peoples and communities?

Conclusion

Healthcare services in Australia are generally based on Western frameworks of health. These frameworks do not address the health and wellbeing needs of Aboriginal and Torres Strait Islander peoples as they do not align with their holistic view of health based on cultural values, beliefs and traditions passed down over generations. For Aboriginal and Torres Strait Islander peoples, a person's health and wellbeing is impacted by connection to family, kin, community, country, culture, spirituality and ancestors. As the biomedical, the biopsychosocial and the ICF frameworks are reductionist in nature, they do not account for the complex interplay of a multitude of factors that impact on health and social and emotional wellbeing; that is, they do not foster a holistic approach to healthcare.

SUMMARY

Throughout this chapter you have been encouraged to reflect on how healthcare services in Australia are generally based on Western frameworks of health. You have considered how these frameworks do not address the health and wellbeing needs of Aboriginal and Torres Strait Islander peoples as they do not align with their holistic view of health based on cultural values, beliefs and traditions passed down over generations.

Learning concept 1

Identify differences between Western and Aboriginal and Torres Strait Islander peoples' concepts of health and social and emotional wellbeing: For Aboriginal and Torres Strait Islander peoples, a person's health and wellbeing is impacted by connection to family, kin, community, country, culture, spirituality and ancestors.

Learning concept 2

Explain the biomedical, biopsychosocial, ICF and socio-ecological frameworks of health and wellbeing: The biomedical framework of healthcare is based on the premise that there are two states—a healthy state and an ill state. The biopsychosocial framework proposes that health is determined by the dynamic interaction of a person's body structures and functions, subjective behaviours, beliefs, thought processes, motivations and experiences, and culture, family, community and society. The ICF states that health exists along a continuum, rather than being a static state fixed in time, and is a result of dynamic interactions between the person and the environment. The socio-ecological framework encourages a social justice approach to practice and acknowledges that health and wellbeing are influenced by factors that operate at the individual, interpersonal, community and societal levels.

Learning concept 3

Discuss the conflict of applying Western frameworks of health and wellbeing to health service delivery for Aboriginal and Torres Strait Islander peoples: Western frameworks are reductionist in nature as they are not holistic and do not account for the complex interplay of a multitude of factors that impact on health and social and emotional wellbeing.

Learning concept 4

Evaluate the interdependent connections between the seven domains comprising the model of social and emotional wellbeing for Aboriginal and Torres Strait Islander peoples: Aboriginal and Torres Strait Islander peoples' understanding of health and wellbeing is based on the interdependent connections between the seven domains (body; mind and emotions; family and kinship; community; culture; country; and spirit, spirituality and ancestors) and on the historical and socio-political determinants that create intergenerational trauma.

Learning concept 5

<u>Discuss the factors that inform effective provision of health and wellbeing services to Aboriginal and Torres Strait Islander peoples:</u> The most effective healthcare for Aboriginal and Torres Strait Islander peoples is offered by Aboriginal Community Controlled Health Services (ACCHSs) as these services are community owned and controlled, employ clinical and managerial Aboriginal staff, implement models of care that embrace Aboriginal knowledge systems, and promote dignity, self-esteem and self-determination. Non-Indigenous health services and professionals should ensure delivery of culturally safe and relevant services to Aboriginal and Torres Strait Islander peoples by embedding a social justice approach and applying the nine guiding principles of the social and emotional wellbeing framework to their practice.

REVISION QUESTIONS

1. What is the difference between Indigenous health and Western frameworks of health?
2. Why are Aboriginal Community Controlled Health Services so important for health and wellbeing?

FURTHER READINGS/ADDITIONAL RESOURCES

Albury Wodonga Aboriginal Health Service: https://www.awahs.com.au

National Aboriginal Community Controlled Health Organisation: https://www.naccho.org.au

Orange Aboriginal Medical Service: https://www.oams.net.au

REFERENCES

Ah Chee, D., Boffa, J., & Tilton, E. (2016). Towards an integrated model for child and family services in central Australia. *Medical Journal of Australia*, 205(1), 8.

Alford, V., Remedios, L., Webb, G., & Ewen, S. (2013). The use of the international classification of functioning, disability and health (ICF) in indigenous healthcare: A systematic literature review. *International Journal for Equity in Health*, 12(32). doi:10.1186/1475-9276-12-32

Australian Institute of Health and Welfare. (2014). *Australia's health 2014*. Australia's health series No. 14, Cat. No. AUS 178. Canberra: AIHW.

Bailie, J., Matthews, V., Laycock, A., Schultz, R., Burgess, C. P., Peiris, D., ... Bailie, R. (2017). Improving preventive health care in Aboriginal and Torres Strait Islander primary care settings. *Globalization & Health*, *13*, 1-13. doi:10.1186/s12992-017-0267-z

Bickenbach, J. (2014). Reconciling the capability approach and the ICF. *Alter, European Journal of Disability Research*, *8*, 10-23. doi:org/10.1016/j.alter.2013.11.005

Blignault, I., & Williams, M. (2017). Challenges in evaluating Aboriginal healing programs: Definitions, diversity and data. *Evaluation Journal of Australasia*, *17*(2), 4-10.

Caffery, L. J., Bradford, N. K., Wickramasinghe, S. I., Hayman, N., & Smith, A. C. (2017). Outcomes of using telehealth for the provision of healthcare to Aboriginal and Torres Strait Islander people: A systematic review. *Australian and New Zealand Journal of Public Health*, *41*(1), 48-53. doi:10.1111/1753-6405.12600

Calma, T., Dudgeon, P., & Bray, A. (2017). Aboriginal and Torres Strait Islander social and emotional wellbeing and mental health. *Australian Psychologist*, *52*(4), 255-260. doi:10.1111/ap.12299

Casey, W. (2014). Strong spirit, strong mind model: Informing policy and practice. In P. Dudgeon, H. Milroy & R. Walker (Eds.), *Working together: Aboriginal and Torres Strait Islander mental health and wellbeing principles and practice* (2nd ed., pp. 449-458). Canberra: Commonwealth of Australia.

Commonwealth of Australia. (2017). *National strategic framework for Aboriginal and Torres Strait Islander peoples' mental health and social and emotional wellbeing*. Canberra: Department of the Prime Minister and Cabinet.

Conti-Becker, A. (2009). Between the ideal and the real: Reconsidering the International Classification of Functioning, Disability and Health. *Disability and Rehabilitation*, *31*(25), 2125-2129.

Davy, C., Kite, E., Aitken, G., Dodd, G., Rigney, J., Hayes, J., & Van Emden, J. (2016). What keeps you strong? A systematic review identifying how primary health-care and aged-care services can support the well-being of older indigenous peoples. *Australasian Journal on Ageing*, *35*(2), 90-97.

Day, A., & Francisco, A. (2013). Social and emotional wellbeing in Indigenous Australians: Identifying promising interventions. *Australian and New Zealand Journal of Public Health*, *37*(4), 350-355. doi:10.1111/1753-6405.12083

Duckett, S. (2007). *The Australian health care system* (3rd ed.). Melbourne: Oxford University Press.

Dudgeon, P., Purdie, N., Walker, R., & Calma, T. (Eds.). (2014). *Working together: Aboriginal and Torres Strait Islander mental health and wellbeing principles and practice* (2nd ed.). Canberra: Australian Government Department of the Prime Minister and Cabinet.

Dwyer, J., O'Donnell, K., Willis, E., & Kelly, J. (2016). Equitable care for Indigenous people: Every health service can do it. *Asia Pacific Journal of Health Management*, *11*(3), 11-17.

Fisher, M., Baum, F., Kay, A., & Frie, S. (2017). Are changes in Australian national primary healthcare policy likely to promote or impede equity of access? A narrative review. *Australian Journal of Primary Health*, *23*(3), 209-215. doi:10.1071/PY16152

Foster, M. (2008). Fields of health service provision. In S. Taylor, M. Foster & J. Fleming (Eds.), *Health care practice in Australia: Policy, context and innovation* (pp. 74-102). Melbourne: Oxford University Press.

Foster, M., & Fleming, J. (2008). The policy context of health care practice. In S. Taylor, M. Foster & J. Fleming (Eds.), *Health care practice in Australia: Policy, context and innovations* (pp. 131-160). Melbourne: Oxford University Press.

Francis-Cracknell, A., Gilby, R., & Adams, K. (2017). Teaching innovations: Collaborative academic strengthening in Indigenous health. An interdisciplinary experience. In *LIME good practice case studies volume 4* (pp. 46-51). Melbourne: Onemda VicHealth Koori Health Unit, University of Melbourne.

Gee, G., Dudgeon, P., Schultz, C., Hart, A., & Kelly, K. (2014). Aboriginal and Torres Strait Islander social and emotional wellbeing. In P. Dudgeon, H. Milroy & R. Walker (Eds.), *Working together: Aboriginal and Torres Strait Islander mental health and wellbeing principles and practice*. Canberra: Australian Government Department of the Prime Minister and Cabinet.

Germov, J. (2018). Imagining health problems as social issues. In J. Germov (Ed.), *Second opinion: An introduction to health sociology* (6th ed., pp. 5-22). Melbourne: Oxford University Press.

Gillen, A., & Greber, C. (2014). Occupation-focused practice: Challenges and choices. *British Journal of Occupational Therapy*, 77(1), 39-41. doi:10.4276/030802214X13887685335580

Gilroy, J., Dew, A., Lincoln, M., & Hines, M. (2017). Need for an Australian Indigenous disability workforce strategy: Review of the literature. *Disability & Rehabilitation*, 39(16), 1664-1673. doi:10.1080/09638288.2016.1201151

Gilroy, J., Donelly, M., Colmar, S., & Parmenter, T. (2013). Conceptual framework for policy and research development with Indigenous peoples with disabilities. *Australian Aboriginal Studies*, 2, 42-58.

Gomersall, J. S., Gibson, O., Dwyer, J., O'Donnell, K., Stephenson, M., Carter, D., ... Brown, A. (2017). What Indigenous Australian clients value about primary health care: A systematic review of qualitative evidence. *Australian & New Zealand Journal of Public Health*, 41(4), 417-423. doi:10.1111/1753-6405.12687

Gormon, D., Nielsen, A., & Best, O. (2006). Western medicine and Australian Indigenous healing practices. *Aboriginal and Islander Health Worker Journal*, 30(1), 28-29.

Hemmingsson, H., & Jonsson, H. (2005). An occupational perspective on the concept of participation in the International Classification of Functioning, Disability and Health: Some critical remarks. *American Journal of Occupational Therapy*, 59(5569-5576).

Hill, S., Ewen, S. C., Paul, D., & Wilkin, A. (2017). Can my mechanic fix blue cars? A discussion of health clinicians' interactions with Aboriginal Australian clients. *Australian Journal of Rural Health*, 25(3), 189-192. doi:10.1111/ajr.12299

Hocking, C. (2013). Occupation for public health. *New Zealand Journal of Occupational Therapy*, 60(1), 33-37.

Hume Chambers, A., & Walker, R. (2012). Introduction to health promotion. In P. Liamputtong, R. Fanany & G. Verrinder (Eds.), *Health, illness and well-being* (pp. 107-124). Melbourne: Oxford University Press.

Isbel, S., & Jamieson, M. (2017). An overview of the Australian health care system. In T. Brown, H. Bourke-Taylor, S. Isbel & R. Cordier (Eds.), *Occupational therapy in Australia: Professional and practice issues* (pp. 14-26). Melbourne: Allen & Unwin.

Jackson King, J., & Dender, A. (2017). Indigenous health: Occupational therapy's role. In T. Brown, H. Bourke-Taylor, S. Isbel & R. Cordier (Eds.), *Occupational therapy in Australia: Professional and practice issues* (pp. 331-338). Melbourne: Allen & Unwin.

Jirojwong, S., & Liamputtong, P. (2009a). Introduction: Population health and health promotion. In S. Jirojwong & P. Liamputtong (Eds.), *Population health, communities and health promotion* (pp. 3-25). Melbourne: Oxford University Press.

Jirojwong, S., & Liamputtong, P. (2009b). Primary health care and health promotion. In S. Jirojwong & P. Liamputtong (Eds.), *Population health, communities and health promotion* (pp. 26-42). Melbourne: Oxford University Press.

Kendall, E., Milliken, J., Barnet, L., & Marshall, C. (2008). Improving practice by respecting Indigenous knowledge and ways of knowing. In S. Taylor, M. Foster & J. Fleming (Eds.), *Health care practice in Australia: Policy, context and innovations* (pp. 220-238). Melbourne: University of Oxford.

King, R. (2014). The experience of flow and meaningful occupation. In K. Jacobs, N. MacRae & K. Sladyk (Eds.), *Occupational therapy essentials for clinical competence* (pp. 3-10). Thorofare: SLACK Incorporated.

Le Grande, M., Ski, C., Thompson, D., Scuffham, P., Kularatna, S., Jackson, A., & Brown, A. (2017). Social and emotional wellbeing assessment instruments for use with Indigenous Australians: A critical review. *Social Science & Medicine, 187*, 164-173. doi:http://dx.doi.org/10.1016/j.socscimed.2017.06.046

Liamputtong, P., Fanany, R., & Verrinder, G. (2012). Health, illness, and well-being: An introduction. In P. Liamputtong, R. Fanany & G. Verrinder (Eds.), *Health, illness and well-being* (pp. 1-17). Melbourne: Oxford University Press.

Lindeman, M., Mackell, P., Lin, X., Farthing, A., Jensen, H., Meredith, M., & Haralambous, B. (2017). Role of art centres for Aboriginal Australians living with dementia in remote communities. *Australasian Journal on Ageing, 36*(2), 128-133.

McCalman, J., Bainbridge, R., Percival, N., & Tsey, K. (2016). The effectiveness of implementation in Indigenous Australian healthcare: An overview of literature reviews. *International Journal for Equity in Health, 15*, 1-13. doi:10.1186/s12939-016-0337-5

McFarlane, K., Devine, S., Judd, J., Nichols, N., & Watt, K. (2017). Workforce insights on how health promotion is practised in an Aboriginal Community Controlled Health Service. *Australian Journal of Primary Health, 23*(3), 243-248. doi:10.1071/PY16033

Moll, S., Gewurtz, R., Krupa, T., & Law, M. (2013). Promoting an occupational perspective in public health. *Canadian Journal of Occupational Therapy, 80*(2), 111-119. doi:10.1177/0008417413482271

National Aboriginal Health Strategy Working Party. (1989). *A national Aboriginal health strategy*. Canberra: Commonwealth of Australia.

Peterson, D., Mpofu, E., & Oakland, T. (2010). Concepts and models in disability, functioning, and health. In E. Mpofu & T. Oakland (Eds.), *Rehabilitation and health assessment: Applying ICF guidelines* (pp. 3-26). New York: Springer Publishing Company.

Priest, N., Thompson, L., Mackean, T., Baker, A., & Waters, E. (2017). 'Yarning up with Koori kids'—hearing the voices of Australian urban Indigenous children about their health and well-being. *Ethnicity & Health*, *22*(6), 631-647. doi:10.1080/13557858.2016.1246418

Rumbold, B., & Dickson-Swift, V. (2012). Social determinants of health: Historical developments and global implications. In P. Liamputtong, R. Fanany & G. Verrinder (Eds.), *Health, illness and well-being* (pp. 177-196). Melbourne: Oxford University Press.

Schultz, R., & Cairney, S. (2017). Caring for country and the health of Aboriginal and Torres Strait Islander Australians. *Medical Journal of Australia*, *207*(1), 8-10. doi:10.5694/mja16.00687

Social Health Reference Group. (2004). *Social and emotional well being framework: A national strategic framework for Aboriginal and Torres Strait Islander peoples' mental health and social and emotional well being 2004–2009*. Canberra: National Aboriginal and Torres Strait Islander Health Council and National Mental Health Working Group.

Stewart, J. M., Sanson-Fisher, R. W., Eades, S., & Fitzgerald, M. (2012). The risk status, screening history and health concerns of Aboriginal and Torres Strait Islander people attending an aboriginal community controlled health service. *Drug and Alcohol Review*, *31*(5), 617-624.

Taket, A. (2012). Health and social justice. In P. Liamputtong, R. Fanany & G. Verrinder (Eds.), *Health, illness and well-being* (pp. 278-301). Melbourne: Oxford University Press.

Taylor, S. (2008a). The concept of health. In S. Taylor, M. Foster & J. Fleming (Eds.), *Health care practice in Australia: Policy, context and innovations* (pp. 3-21). Melbourne: Oxford University Press.

Taylor, S. (2008b). Contemporary frameworks of health care. In S. Taylor, M. Foster & J. Fleming (Eds.), *Health care practice in Australia: Policy, context and innovations* (pp. 22-45). Melbourne: Oxford University Press.

Thomas, S., Williams, K., Ritchie, J., & Zwi, K. (2015). Improving paediatric outreach services for urban Aboriginal children through partnerships: Views of community-based service providers. *Child: Care, Health and Development*, *41*(6), 836-842.

Thompson, G., Talley, N. J., & Kong, K. M. (2017). The health of Indigenous Australians. *Medical Journal of Australia*, *207*(1), 19-20. doi:10.5694/mja17.00381

Thorpe, A., Arabena, K., Sullivan, P., Silburn, K., & Rowley, K. (2016). *Engaging first peoples: A review of government engagement methods for developing health policy*. Melbourne: The Lowitja Institute.

Tsey, K., Whiteside, M., Haswell-Elkins, M., Bainbridge, R., Cadet-James, Y., & Wilson, A. (2010). Empowerment and indigenous Australian health: A synthesis of findings from family wellbeing formative research. *Health & Social Care in the Community*, *18*(2), 169-179.

United Nations. (1948). *Universal Declaration of Human Rights*. Retrieved from http://www.un.org/en/universal-declaration-human-rights/index.html

Wakerman, J., & Shannon, C. (2016). Strengthening primary health care to improve Indigenous health outcomes. *Medical Journal of Australia*, *10*(6 June), 363-364. doi:10.5694/mja16.00031

Ward, R., & Gorman, D. (2010). Racism, discrimination and health services to Aboriginal people in south west Queensland. *Aboriginal and Islander Health Worker Journal*, *34*(6), 3-5.

Ware, V. (2013). *Improving the accessibility of health services in urban and regional settings for Indigenous people: Resource sheet no. 27.* Canberra: Closing the Gap Clearinghouse, Australian Government, AIHW, AIFS. Retrieved from https://www.aihw.gov.au/getmedia/186eb114-8fc8-45cc-acef-30f6d05a9c0c/ctgc-rs27.pdf.aspx?inline=true

Whalley Hammell, K. (2004). Deviating from the norm: A skeptical interrogation of the classificatory practice of the ICF. *British Journal of Occupational Therapy, 67*(9), 408-411.

Whalley Hammell, K., & Iwama, M. (2012). Well-being and occupational rights: An imperative for critical occupational therapy. *Scandinavian Journal of Occupational Therapy, 19*(5), 385-394. doi:10.3109/11038128.2011.611821

Wilcock, A., & Hocking, C. (2015). *An occupational perspective of health* (3rd ed.). Thorofare: SLACK Incorporated.

Wilson, A. M., Kelly, J., Magarey, A., Jones, M., & Mackean, T. (2016). Working at the interface in Aboriginal and Torres Strait Islander health: Focussing on the individual health professional and their organisation as a means to address health equity. *International Journal for Equity in Health, 15*, 1-12. doi:10.1186/s12939-016-0476-8

World Health Organization. (1948). Preamble. *Constitution of the World Health Organization* (p. 1). Retrieved from http://www.who.int/about/mission/en/

World Health Organization. (1978). *Primary health care: Report of the International Conference on Primary Health Care.* Alma-Ata, USSR, 6-12 September 1978. Retrieved from http://apps.who.int/iris/handle/10665/39228.

World Health Organization. (2001). *International classification of functioning, disability and health (ICF).* Fifty-fourth World Health Assembly, May 2001. Retrieved from http://www.who.int/classifications/icf/en/

World Health Organization. (2011). *Rio declaration on social determinants of health.* Presented at World Conference on Social Determinants of Health, Rio de Janeiro, Brazil. Retrieved from http://www.who.int/sdhconference/declaration/Rio_political_declaration.pdf?ua=1

World Health Organization. (2013). *Health in all policies.* Paper presented at the 8th Global Conference on Health Promotion, Helsinki, Finland. Retrieved from http://www.who.int/healthpromotion/conferences/8gchp/statement_2013/en/

World Health Organization, Health and Welfare Canada, & Canadian Public Health Association. (1986). *Ottawa charter for health promotion.* Ottawa: World Health Organization.

CHAPTER **FOUR**

Aboriginal and Torres Strait Islander health research champions: A snapshot

Brett Biles, James Charles and Jessica Biles

LEARNING CONCEPTS

Studying this chapter should enable you to:

1. develop some understanding of Aboriginal and Torres Strait Islander health research.
2. explore ethical research principles relevant to Aboriginal and Torres Strait Islander health research.
3. identify the key aspects of Aboriginal and Torres Strait Islander research processes.
4. explore Aboriginal and Torres Strait Islander research methodologies.
5. explore examples of key Aboriginal and Torres Strait Islander research champions.

KEY TERMS

community
Dadirri
holistic
methodology
reciprocity
yarning

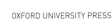

74   Part 1: Frameworks for health and competence

Introduction

This chapter will encourage you to reflect and consider Aboriginal and Torres Strait Islander research. This will involve exploration of the history of this research, ethical principles related to Aboriginal and Torres Strait Islander research, the research process, the foundational exploration of methodologies and a snapshot of contemporary Aboriginal and Torres Strait Islander health research champions. This chapter will combine both traditional and non-traditional forms of writing. Some aspects of this chapter will be written work that is supported by literature; others will involve conversational language. As we developed this chapter we held a number of '**yarning** sessions' that brought to life the research process from an Aboriginal viewpoint. Importantly, these yarns will add depth to your understanding of Aboriginal and Torres Strait Islander research.

yarning A term used by Aboriginal and Torres Strait Islander people to mean a conversation or dialogue between Aboriginal and Torres Strait Islander people.

Historically, the majority of Indigenous-related research has been carried out by non-Indigenous people and has not been a positive experience for many Aboriginal and Torres Strait Islander communities (Smith, 1999). Researchers have a responsibility to cause no harm, but traditional forms of research frequently have been a source of distress for Aboriginal and Torres Strait Islander peoples due to inappropriate methods and practices (Cochran et al., 2008).

Ethical research principles within Aboriginal and Torres Strait Islander peoples' health research

This section will briefly discuss the historical aspect of Indigenous research and the key aspects involved in ethical research with Aboriginal and Torres Strait Islander peoples. It will also touch on a few peak bodies relating to state- and national-based Indigenous research.

Ethical considerations

> **Brett**   We are going to yarn about the Aboriginal Health and Medical Health Research Council (AH&MRC) or state equivalent, and the Australian Institute of Aboriginal and Torres Strait Islander Studies (AIATSIS). AH&MRC and AIATSIS produced guidelines for conducting ethical research with Aboriginal and Torres Strait Islander peoples. So James,

can you give us a bit of a brief introduction around why these guidelines first came out?

James The guidelines were produced because there has been a lot of inappropriate, unnecessary, biased research that probably doesn't have the benefit of the Indigenous **community** in mind. Also a lack of consultation with Indigenous people, so some of the guidelines enforce or ensure that the communities' best interest[s] are in [the] mind[s] of researchers and that the Indigenous individuals and communities involved have some control over what research is taking place.

community A group of people living in the same place, sharing and having similar interests and attitudes in common.

Brett So just before we go into the 14 principles that AIATSIS produced, let's set the scene. The principles are about giving Aboriginal people inherent rights, and that includes the right to self-determination and [that] the ethical guidelines are based on respect for these rights. That's the right to full and fair participation in any processes, projects and activities that impact on Indigenous people and the right to maintain our culture and heritage. It's really important that we consider [that] these principles are not only a matter of ethical research practice but are ethical human rights. I think what is really important is that as Aboriginal people we have to maintain full participation within any research that is pertaining to us as Indigenous people. We have to share and understand the aims and methods of the research. It's not just writing about us, but researchers have to involve us in the process, and share the results of the work. It needs to be transparent at every stage of the research, prior to getting ethics approval. It's community consultation; being involved on advisory groups at each phase. We need to be involved through meaningful consultation and engagement. This is also about reciprocity between the researcher and Indigenous people. So from a reciprocity perspective, can you give an example of what that actually means?

James **Reciprocity** is about giving back and sharing, not just taking. A lot of Aboriginal and Torres Strait Islander peoples' cultures are about giving and sharing, and that is a really important part of culture. So anyone wanting to conduct research needs to understand that it is about giving, sharing and about having equal partnerships— everyone having a role in the community, and a level of control in the community. That is why it is important for universities or researchers and the community to have that equal sharing and working in partnership, within written formal agreements; with Memorandums of Understanding to put all those things in place. Like we will be

reciprocity A practice of exchange that yields mutual benefits.

equal and that we will be sharing, and that any group can choose not to participate in any area that they don't want to. That's an important part of any research to have that included—perhaps right from the very beginning to have a formal agreement so that everyone knows and understands the rights of both sides.

Brett   I think if you use those words, 'equal partners', it is very important—it means we are all on the same playing field.

James   Yes, it's crucial, as this has not been the case in the past.

Brett   So from a non-Aboriginal perspective, from a research perspective, Aboriginal people are part of the research and they are researchers as well. So we need to be involved from the get-go, until the absolute finished project; having a clear understanding, having a say, knowing exactly what is going to happen with the research data and outcomes.

AIATSIS has 14 key principles that can be grouped under six broad categories [see Table 4.1]. When we go on to discuss the Aboriginal Health and Medical Research Council from a NSW perspective, there is some overlap with these 14 guiding principles but from a health research domain.

I'd like to have a bit of a yarn around advisory groups. James, can you talk about your experience around why advisory groups are important?

James   It's about the knowledge, experience and understanding what Indigenous individuals and communities own and what they will share to guide the researcher. Even some Indigenous people may not fully understand the local sensitivities and that's why it is important to have a local advisory group, as opposed to any advisory group. Ideally, the members of the advisory group will be involved with the local community, perhaps involved at some level with the local community control organisation. It is fine to have other advisors, like individuals that are at a government department or a university. However, it is much more important that you have that local knowledge and understanding of the cultural sensitivities of the local community, who know how to contact people in that community and how to follow up those people to share information. An advisory group is also designed to protect the rights of the Indigenous community involved with the research, and protect the researcher. If you don't have that advisory group or some kind of committee that is informing research, then really you are trampling the rights of Indigenous people. It is about respecting culture and then doing research in a sensitive way. So in a lot of ways it is just being respectful, and not circumventing

Table 4.1 AIATSIS Principles for Ethical Research in Australian Indigenous Studies

Category	Principle
1. Rights, respect and recognition	1. Recognition of the diversity and uniqueness of peoples, as well as of individuals, is essential.
	2. The rights of Indigenous peoples to self-determination must be recognised.
	3. The rights of Indigenous peoples to their intangible heritage must be recognised.
	4. Rights in the traditional knowledge and traditional cultural expressions of Indigenous peoples must be respected, protected and maintained.
	5. Indigenous knowledge, practices and innovations must be respected, protected and maintained.
2. Negotiation, consultation, agreement and mutual understanding	6. Consultation, negotiation and free, prior and informed consent are the foundations for research with or about Indigenous peoples.
	7. Responsibility for consultation and negotiation is ongoing.
	8. Consultation and negotiation should achieve mutual understanding about the proposed research.
	9. Negotiation should result in a formal agreement for the conduct of a research project.
3. Participation, collaboration and partnership	10. Indigenous people have the right to full participation appropriate to their skills and experiences in research projects and processes.
4. Benefits, outcomes and giving back	11. Indigenous people involved in research, or who may be affected by research, should benefit from, and not be disadvantaged by, the research project.
	12. Research outcomes should include specific results that respond to the needs and interests of Indigenous people.
5. Managing research: use, storage and access	13. Plans should be agreed for managing use of, and access to, research results.
6. Reporting and compliance	14. Research projects should include appropriate mechanisms and procedures for reporting on ethical aspects of the research and complying with these guidelines.

Source: Australian Institute of Aboriginal and Torres Strait Islander Studies (2012).

community control—say, for example, by going to a government department and talking to an Indigenous person that may not be from that community, who may not have the local understanding and may not know the community involved.

Jess   So do you think that working parties and special interest groups would be a good start for somebody that is not part of the community?

James   Yes, I think that's a great place to start, and that is all part of it—a lot of the Indigenous people on those committees are often part of the community. So I think the local Aboriginal Education Consultative Group have all sections of NSW covered, so they can put you in the right direction. However, you need to get that Memorandum of Understanding with a local Aboriginal-controlled organisation above and beyond that.

Brett   Yes, and [this touches] back on to the AH&MRC principles as well as cultural sensitivity. The rights of local Indigenous people too, because we are diverse and uniquely different.

Jess   So I am confused with the principles of AIATSIS and AH&MRC. If I am a researcher in NSW, am I bound by both?

Brett   No. If you are a researcher in health in NSW you are bound by the AH&MRC principles. Research in general, if it is not health-related, you would be going through the AIATSIS principles.

Key aspects of Aboriginal and Torres Strait Islander health research

There is an interrelationship between the three key processes of community participation, lengthy process and engagement. Each element is dependent on the others and will be discussed in a piecemeal way.

Community participation

Brett   James can you give some of the reasons and rationales around why the Aboriginal Health and Medical Research Council (AH&MRC) first came about?

James Similar to AIATSIS, in health, historically a lot of research being conducted was inappropriate, unnecessary and not from an Indigenous perspective either. Researchers were looking at research from a really Western arbitrary point of view, in a lot of ways looking to blame, at least from that perspective—like, 'Indigenous health is not good', but it could not be due to colonisation or poor policy, and looking for evidence to only blame Indigenous people. Researchers would say, 'Oh they don't do this and they don't do that and here's our evidence that supports that is why they have health problems' and this is the only reason their health is bad. It really should be recognised that poor health may be a symptom; for example, [of] oppression. The reasons for the AH&MRC ethics committees is to try and scrutinise in more detail what researchers are doing, what they are investigating and why they are investigating it. I can give you an example of a poor approach to Indigenous health research. When I was working in Muna Paiendi in Adelaide, we would get a lot of researchers coming and asking for approval to do research. At our team meetings we would discuss requests [and] sometimes we would ask researchers to come and present to our staff. I remember a staff member asked, 'Why do you want to do this research?' The researcher said, 'Oh well, I just got some funding so I thought I would come and do it.' The staff member just got up and walked out. The researcher had absolutely no respect or real interest in the wellbeing of Indigenous people. All the staff walked away just shaking our heads going, 'Oh my god, I can't believe some researchers have no sensitivity or empathy, and are only interested in their own development.'

Brett I think what is really paramount is the AH&MRC have these five key principles around research. And when you submit your ethics application to the AH&MRC, you actually have to address these five key principles. The [first principle is] net benefits for Indigenous people and communities. The second is the Indigenous control of research, and I think that second one is extremely important. Because from a control perspective, we always have that aspect around. So [when] we are researching, from a general Western perspective or paradigm we 'own' the data, when in fact, non-Indigenous people (or even we as Indigenous people who are doing research around Indigenous people) [shouldn't] own the research. The communities own the research and they have the final say into how, when and where it is used. The third key point is around cultural sensitivity, and the fourth one is around reimbursements of costs, which at times can challenge people's perspectives of what that actually means. The last one, which I think is absolutely paramount, is enhancing Indigenous peoples' skills and knowledge, which is around leaving that legacy of empowering people and allowing self-determination. It is about making sure that we are leaving a positive aspect around enhancing skills and knowledges.

Can you tell us about how we look at addressing the net benefits for Indigenous individuals and communities?

James Yeah, I think that's the problem. Some academics just see Indigenous research as an opportunity to get a PhD or funding to do some research without any consideration for the Aboriginal and Torres Strait Islander communities' wellbeing. I think any research needs to have outcomes that have some net benefit for the community, like assisting the community to get more funding for things that are lacking, like better facilities. I have been to a lot of small communities with tiny Aboriginal Medical Services where they have got nothing more than a small hall as a part-time clinic and not really much more than that, and of course this lack of infrastructure impacts on health. A lot of people think, 'Oh, Aboriginal and Torres Strait Islander communities get so much funding', but my experience on the ground is that is not the case. So researchers need to go to communities for the right reasons, with the benefit of the community paramount. Aboriginal and Torres Strait Islander communities need translational research to discover better ways to operate, or more appropriate clinical approaches, and not the use of the data collected against the communities.

Lengthy process

Brett Yeah, [I] agree and would like to add that when you are looking at what those net benefits are, it's around having tangible outcomes, and I think that is really important. There was some research done back in 1999 by Voyle and Simmons and they were saying that programs that are aimed at improving Indigenous health should include program and development, appointment of community-based liaison workers—i.e. Aboriginal health workers—and the formation of partnership committees as well. So it is more about Indigenous people having a strong voice within any decision around what's going on within their particular community. So you have that empowerment from the ground up, and it's that self-determination. Anyone coming here doing a PhD project, you are not just ticking the box because you want to get these initials after your name. It's not about that; it's about us as Indigenous researchers having that link to our community, being part of that voice for our community, needing to get that Indigenous voice shining through. I think for us Indigenous researchers it can be a challenge at times because we are part of the community as well. But for Indigenous people, as well as non-Indigenous researchers, coming in to that particular space as well, it does take time.

James   Oh yes, it does take time, and it can't be rushed. It does take a lot of time and a lot of long-term commitment. This is needed, and needs to be demonstrated before an Aboriginal Health Service will sign off on doing any form of research. I think that is a really good segue into the second aspect, which is around Indigenous community control of research, and what that actually means.

Brett   Can you give us a few examples of what Indigenous control of research actually means and what it looks like? Because it can be very challenging for non-Indigenous researchers to fully understand.

James   A lot of it is about the mistrust from inappropriate research that has happened in the past. The Indigenous 'voice' needs to be heard and researchers need to listen actively, that is why engagement is so important. It is about the empowerment of the Indigenous community, to give people control over what's happening. A lot of Aboriginal Medical Services have their own ethics committee to empower the local community, which overrides any other approvals. The local community themselves can still say 'no' or 'we want this changed'. This is a ground-up approach to power, as opposed to top-down, giving the local community control over what is happening.

Brett   Yes, [I] agree. If you are looking for an actual reference, McMurray [2003, p. 296] defines goals for Indigenous health as 'inclusive of access and equity in healthcare, greater connectivity between Indigenous peoples and their advocates', which is really important, and [also highlights] 'cultural sensitivity, cultural safety in all healthcare practices' [and] 'community self-determination, self-empowerment on the basis of capacity building'. So you, as an Indigenous person, owning that particular research; having control of that research [so] you can shape where that research is taking you and your community, which is absolutely paramount. This really challenges the status quo; that Western paradigm of what research really is. In some areas of research in the Western paradigm, research is commercially driven. It is paramount that Aboriginal and Torres Strait Islander peoples have ownership and control in all facets of research. Therefore, commercially driven research in Aboriginal and Torres Strait Islander communities can have many complex considerations. I think from a strengths-based approach, having that community control of research, is really adding to us as Indigenous people and is enhancing our knowledge and our skills.

James   Well, it sort of links back to that net benefit. If the community can control and own the data and control what's published, they have the power to say 'no'—what you are writing here is not what we are saying. So ensuring the first key point about the net benefits for the individuals and for the community is maintained. If the community have ownership of all data, then they can ensure it's used appropriately, as opposed to people going away and using that data however they see fit, which might not necessarily be in the best interests of the community.

Engagement

Brett   Why it is important to address those key issues around what is cultural sensitivity, and what that looks like from an ethical aspect?

James   I think part of cultural sensitivity is around [the fact that] we as Indigenous people are so diverse, and often people think there is one group of Aboriginal and Torres Strait Islander people and we are all the same. The sensitivity around that is that we as Indigenous individuals—we don't know it all. And just because we are Indigenous, people shouldn't assume we have all the answers. Obviously, we don't know everything around all Indigenous peoples. I think from a research perspective we need to make sure that when we are researching Indigenous peoples that, before we even start the journey of research, local Indigenous peoples are involved in research, from pre setting up our research proposal, ethics applications, throughout our whole journey. And making sure the Indigenous peoples' voice is coming through what we are writing and what we are presenting. Also knowing that we as researchers might have one key aspect that we want to focus on, but for the community it might not be required. So as researchers, we need to make sure that we are fluid and flexible; for example, the researcher might say, 'Yes we have four key questions we want answered', but from community consultation and engagement you may find that the community has a completely different view and approach. Therefore, as the researcher you need to be an active listener to the community's needs.

Jess So as a non-Indigenous researcher, how would I go about setting up those relationships?

Brett Well, I think part of it is that you have to get outside your comfort zone. When we are talking about research, you know, [it] comes in many different ways, shapes and forms. I think building that relationship first and foremost is probably almost outside your research scope, in that it is not really about the research—it's about relationship building. It is about attending local events, for example. Like most Indigenous places, it is quite generic; we tend to have community working party meetings or we will have Aboriginal Education Consultative Groups (AECG) and things like that. It's about being part of it and showing your face there as a person first and foremost—not as Jess, James or Brett from CSU or from some university, but you as a person wanting to be involved with the community. [Also] bearing in mind [that while] people are made to feel welcome ... Indigenous people often have their shutters up and obviously will not welcome you with open arms until they get to know you.

James They are checking you out.

Brett Yes, exactly. Absolutely.

James Do we trust this person.

Brett Exactly.

James I think even clinically a lot of Indigenous people do that as well. When an Indigenous person goes in to see a health professional, they often pause before giving an answer. It might not be because they don't know the answer, [but because] they will be thinking, 'Do I share with this person?' Even something that [the] health professional may think is straightforward, but they might be reluctant to share because they don't trust them. It is important to listen and take time to build that trust and rapport because you need to listen for a while and hear what people are saying and get some understanding.

Brett Absolutely, catching up with the community sort of thing. The Community Working Party meetings, going down to your local

Aboriginal Health Service is really important, but also attending cultural events—like most places have NAIDOC events, Sorry Day events as well—and obviously just being around. People will see you there and might not know who you are at the start, but they will remember you if you continually turn up. Even as an Indigenous researcher, when you are doing research, I think with my project it has taken two to two-and-a-half years to build that trust; for the local guys to tell their story to me. In that safe space as well, because of those historical fears around use and abuse basically of Indigenous peoples' voices.

James   A safe space for Indigenous people is so important, where people are more likely to be comfortable and be more open. My advice would be to go in person to those places, even if not much is happening, [because] that is showing your interest and people will see you. You have to put yourself out there, maybe outside your comfort zone, because if you don't then you are probably not going to get very far. That would be my advice for Indigenous and non-Indigenous people as well. That's why it often doesn't work when people try to invite Indigenous people to participate in research at a university clinic—if Indigenous people don't feel comfortable, they probably won't go. Take your research to the community. It's about inclusiveness, making everyone feel part of the process and building the capacity of those people. I think every project should be saying, 'We are going to invite you', certainly Aboriginal health workers and other community members acting as advisors. To be part of even the collection of the data, or analysing the data, to build that capacity of those Indigenous people. Not just only for that particular research project but [to] have the skills to be involved with other research and with new research skills; for example, analysing, publication or presenting results. I think there is no one better than a community member getting the opportunity to share some of the research that they were part of.

Exploration of Aboriginal and Torres Strait Islander health research methodologies

Methods are important in any research and particularly when involving Aboriginal and Torres Strait Islander peoples. In this section we will briefly start to look at Aboriginal and Torres Strait Islander research methods that are commonly implemented.

Indigenous **methodology** emerged from the Canadian and Native American communities, gaining momentum in Australia in the early 1990s (Rigney, 1997). Fundamentally, Indigenous research methodology decolonises and incorporates an epistemological stance where Indigenous worldviews are the focus and drive the methodological framework (Sherwood, 2010). It has been discussed that Aboriginal and Torres Strait Islander researchers experience a constant struggle between Western views of research and Aboriginal and Torres Strait Islander peoples' views, protocols and cultural considerations regarding research (Laycock, Walker, Harrison & Brands, 2011). As Aboriginal and Torres Strait Islander researchers emerge, we can see methodology and methods that are responsive to cultural protocols, beliefs and traditions (Martin, 2003). Commonly Aboriginal and Torres Strait Islander peoples are at the centre driving these methodologies, with the researcher as an agent of change (Laycock et al., 2011). Methods to decolonise and enable an Aboriginal and Torres Strait Islander peoples' paradigm have been explored by many scholars (Moreton-Robinson, 2017; Nakata, 2007; Rigney, 1997). With this in mind, there are several key methodologies that are used regularly within Australia that bring to life the Aboriginal and Torres Strait Islander research paradigm. As discussed earlier in this chapter, the ethical principles should frame the project and be aligned to a methodology that is responsive to Aboriginal and Torres Strait Islander research principles.

> **methodology** A system of methods used in a particular discipline or area of activity.

The participatory model of research, where the power is held by the participants or decisions are made collaboratively, is well known as a support to effective research in Aboriginal and Torres Strait Islander communities (Baydala, Ruttan & Starkes, 2015). Generally, in participatory methodologies the researcher facilitates the direction the participants deem to be appropriate. There is a significant shift in power between researchers and those researched that enables the research process to respond to community needs (Couzos, Nicholson, Hunt, Davey, May, Bennet & Thomas, 2015). Similarly, action research cycles have been used in Australia as a means to decolonise the research process (Kemmis, McTaggart & Nixon, 2014).

Yarning

As defined by Bessarab and Ng'andu (2010), yarning is a relaxed form of storytelling. As the conversation creates depth, the relationship and trust between the researcher and participants develops. Through this conversation meaning emerges about a topic area. The conversation may involve memories, lived experiences and situations that the participants may share. As discussed by Geia, Hayes and Usher (2013), the researcher must follow some practical steps prior to engaging in a yarning session. These involve preparing well ahead of time and getting to know your participants prior to participating in yarning sessions (Kovach, 2009), developing and maintaining a mutually respectful relationship, participating in the yarning and sharing some of your personal stories, and practising deep listening.

Dadirri

Dadirri Deep listening, observing and maintaining relationships with others.

As defined by Atkinson (2002), **Dadirri** involves listening, observing and maintaining relationships with others. As we have previously discussed, reciprocity is imperative in all facets of Aboriginal and Torres Strait Islander research and Dadirri has been used as a method in Indigenous research (West, Stewart, Foster & Usher, 2012). Dadirri in action has been described as involving 'listening, reflecting, observing feelings and actions' (West et al., p. 1584) in a cyclic process that brings to life the voice of the participants (Atkinson, 2002, p. 15; West et al., 2012).

Given the historical perspectives that have been previously discussed in this chapter, it is critical for the researcher to bring to life the voice of the participant in both qualitative and quantitative research. The following case studies of research champions will highlight ways that a researcher can bring to life the voice of Aboriginal and Torres Strait Islander peoples.

Interestingly, Aboriginal and Torres Strait Islander researchers are often members of the community they are involved with from a research perspective. This has been referred to as being involved in insider research; that is the 'study of one's own social group or society' (Greene, 2014). This creates new and interesting challenges for a researcher. They often have close relationships with research participants and have valuable insights into the research and health needs of a community. This brings to light a new and interesting scenario that involves researchers requiring both the critical thought of an outsider and the sensitivity and maturity to work with a community (Smith, 1999). This involves researchers walking the path of both community member (abiding by family, community and kinship obligations) while also respecting and upholding the values pertinent to a researcher (VicHealth Koori Health Research and Community Development Unit, 2001).

Aboriginal and Torres Strait Islander health research champions—case studies

This section will celebrate a number of key Aboriginal and Torres Strait Islander health research champions. In each case study they will reveal their nation, research area and clinical expertise, and provide advice for undergraduate students considering research with Aboriginal and Torres Strait Islander communities. It is important to note many other key researchers make a unique difference to Aboriginal and Torres Strait Islander peoples' health. They include Professor Juanita Sherwood, Professor Roianne West, Professor Bronwyn Fredricks and Professor Alex Brown. We encourage you to explore all researchers' contributions in more detail.

Associate Professor James Charles

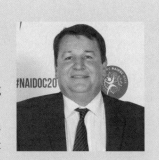

Nation: Kaurna

Role: Associate Professor of Indigenous Teaching and Learning, Deakin University

Research area of interest: Indigenous foot health

Research story: Aboriginal and Torres Strait Islander peoples suffer from high rates of chronic disease, including peripheral vascular disease and diabetes, and the associated increases in morbidity and mortality has an enormous impact on both lifespan and quality of life. Foot health in Aboriginal and Torres Strait Islander peoples is widely accepted to be poor. In those with diabetes, there is a high incidence of neuropathy, foot ulceration, infection and amputation. However, there is little available literature investigating the nature and extent of foot disease in Indigenous peoples, particularly in those with diabetes, or how this can be effectively managed. Anecdotal evidence suggests high rates of restricted ankle joint dorsiflexion (ankle equinus) may exist in the Aboriginal and Torres Strait Islander population, and this may be a significant contributing factor to the development of diabetic foot complications, including pressure ulcerations.

First, selected Aboriginal Community Controlled Health Services (ACCHSs) were consulted and engaged about foot health; that is, Western Sydney Aboriginal Medical Service (Western Sydney), Awabakal Aboriginal Medical Service (Hunter Region) and Tobwabba Aboriginal Medical Service (Mid North Coast). Some board members, staff and community members participated as an advisory group. An Indigenous education centre—the Wollotuka Institute (Newcastle University)—also supported this project. The written support of these organisations was essential for the ethical approval from the Aboriginal Health and Medical Research Council's Ethics Committee.

A literature review was conducted to establish current risk factors and risk markers for poor foot health in Indigenous peoples. Little data were found relating specifically to Indigenous foot health; however, high prevalence of chronic disease associated with foot complications including diabetes, neuropathy and peripheral vascular disease were evident. Lifestyle factors associated with increased risk of chronic disease, including smoking and obesity, were also found to be highly prevalent, particularly in women. No literature investigating the role of lower limb structure or biomechanical function in development of foot complications was found.

It was hypothesised that reduced ankle movement was a contributing factor for Indigenous foot health, so a second review of the literature was conducted

(Continued)

to determine a reliable method of measuring ankle joint range of motion. This review showed significant inconsistency in the literature in relation to the definition and diagnosis of ankle equinus, and a lack of a standardised method for clinical assessment. Based on these findings, a device for accurately measuring ankle equinus was developed, which was established to have excellent inter- and intra-tester reliability.

A culturally appropriate health promotion program for improving foot health, reducing injury and increasing healthy lifestyle choices was developed for the local Worimi Aboriginal community in Forster/Tuncurry, New South Wales. Evaluation of this program demonstrated that it was effective in improving healthy lifestyle knowledge and behaviours, and in reducing risk of lower limb injury. These findings suggest appropriate health promotion may be successful in reducing the risk of foot complications in Indigenous peoples.

Subsequently, two cross-sectional cohort studies, one with Aboriginal and Torres Strait Islander peoples with diabetes and one with Aboriginal and Torres Strait Islander peoples without diabetes, were undertaken to test the hypothesis that restricted ankle joint dorsiflexion increases plantar pressures under the forefoot. High prevalence of isolated gastrocnemius equinus was found in both cohorts. Reducing ankle joint range of dorsiflexion was found to be significantly associated with higher peak pressures under the forefoot, and to be an independent predictor of increasing pressure-time integral under the forefoot in both populations. These results, limited by cross-sectional design, suggest ankle equinus may play a key role in the development of pressure-related forefoot complications in Indigenous peoples.

Visual assessment of Aboriginal skeletal remains of the feet of a small number of Kaurna people and 21,000 year-old footprints of the Paakantji, Ngiyampaa and the Mutthi Mutthi Aboriginal people in Lake Mungo was undertaken. These were examined for arch height, indications of biomechanical characteristics of the foot and ankle, and overt osseous pathology. Many of the ancient footprints showed signs of a high arch foot type similar to modern-day Indigenous footprints. In addition, bony spurring on the calcanei on a number of specimens was consistent with possible restriction in ankle dorsiflexion, suggesting ankle equinus may be an evolutionary trait in this population.

This research used a quantitative method, but a culturally appropriate Aboriginal Musculoskeletal Injury Questionnaire was developed. This questionnaire collected some important information on injury and related pain of participants, but most importantly it gave the participants a 'voice' and a chance to tell the researchers how their injuries were affecting them.

Key message for undergraduate health students: No matter whether you are Indigenous or non-Indigenous, and conducting quantitative, qualitative

Figure 4.1 Aboriginal art, feet health

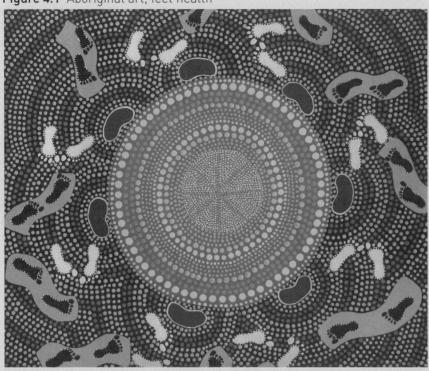

Source: Terry Johnston, *Painting Story of Podiatry Practice and Research*.
Middle circle representing practice, people standing around practice,
footprints around circle showing people coming and going.

or mixed-method research, you must engage and consult with the Indigenous
community involved with the research. Researchers must follow the principles
of ethical research, and incorporate opportunity for the 'voice' of the Indigenous
community to be heard.

Mr Brett Biles

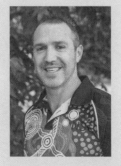

Nation: Murrawarri

Role: Director of Indigenous Health Education in the
Office of Medical Education, UNSW Medicine

Research area of interest: My area of interest is with
Aboriginal men's health and wellbeing, with a key
focus on the effects of exercise and health education
on cardiovascular disease utilising a primary healthcare
approach.

(Continued)

Research story: During my undergraduate degree (physiotherapy), I had no interest in research and could not see the point of the research subjects we had to complete. This could not be further from the truth now, with my doctoral journey coming to an end!

My research can be linked to my family's issues and challenges with cardiovascular disease. My PhD is exploring the effects of a tailored exercise and health-education program on cardiovascular disease for Aboriginal men in a regional setting, by utilising the primary healthcare principles and truly listening to the voices of Aboriginal men. A tailored exercise and health education program was co-created with the local men and implemented to meet their requirements. By truly listening to the needs of the local Aboriginal men and implementing the program they co-created, we were able to achieve an 85% attendance rate for the program.

The data collection for my PhD has ceased, but the exercise program has continued to be conducted over the last 18 months. By clearly listening to the needs of the local Aboriginal men I have been able to honour and privilege their voices, as well as follow another key principle of Aboriginal research, which is reciprocity.

Key message for undergraduate health students: Research is something we do every day in our lives. If you are lucky enough to be involved in Aboriginal research, make sure you truly walk the walk and privilege the voices of Aboriginal people. True community consultation takes time and effort to undertake, but is absolutely paramount in Aboriginal research. And remember you need to follow and implement the key values and principles of Aboriginal research.

Professor Liz Cameron

Nation: Dharug Nation, Murra Murra Clan Group, NSW

Role: Director of the Institute of Koorie Education, Deakin University

Research area of interest: My area of research interest lies within traditional Aboriginal (Dharug) healing practices. This includes Indigenous arts–based therapy, traditional ecologies in land and sea and plants, and preventative and psychological aspects of health.

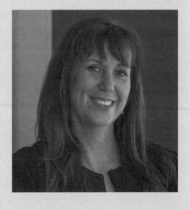

Research story: My research grew out of a concern about the lack of culturally appropriate programs to address health-related issues for Aboriginal people. Unaddressed traumas associated with the impact of colonisation still remain entrenched within contemporary Aboriginal life. Loss and grief is witnessed by historical genocide acts, forced removals of children, dislocations from lands and racial assimilation practices. The prohibitions of cultural and spiritual belief systems have destroyed sustainable living and purpose to life and created dysfunctional communities, exacerbated by the loss of cultural knowledges. As unresolved historical transgenerational trauma continues to impact on Aboriginal health and wellbeing, there is a direct need to reinvigorate traditional healing practices alongside Western scientific ideas to ensure success.

Presently, few programs focus on **holistic** interpretations; that is, those that embed visual literature that communicates cultural meaning and spiritual messages in order to address the physical, emotional and social health of Aboriginal people within a restorative health framework. It has also been identified that there are few culturally traditional sensitive therapeutic initiatives available for Aboriginal people to access, including a lack of long-term sustainable funding. Acknowledgment must also include past, present and future racism, such as the continued stereotypical assumptions that deprive Aboriginal peoples from fulfilling their potential and capabilities.

holistic The idea that parts of a whole are interconnected and interdependent.

Key message for undergraduate health students: Because of past trauma associated with colonisation and present distress associated with situational environmental circumstances, addressing internalised pain and suffering of Aboriginal peoples needs more attention. In recognising traditional Aboriginal healing practices as a valued knowledge system built over thousands of years of life experiences, knowing and appreciating our ways is the first start to positive change. Come, walk with us.

Ms Linda Deravin

Nation: Wiradjuri

Role: Lecturer in Nursing, Charles Sturt University

Research area of interest: Aboriginal and Torres Strait Islander peoples' health policy and how it affects nursing (in progress)

Research story: Government and policy makers have held power and influence over generations of Aboriginal people, which has affected the

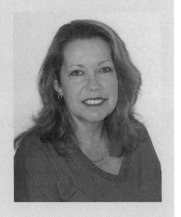

(Continued)

OXFORD UNIVERSITY PRESS

health and wellbeing of this marginalised group. We have seen through history that government-enforced Protection Acts, which resulted in children being taken from their families, were extremely detrimental to Indigenous people. Recognising that social policy had to change, the federal government of Australia in 2008 apologised for the horrific treatment of Aboriginal people and developed the National Partnership Agreement on Closing the Gap in Indigenous Health Outcomes (Council of Australian Governments, 2008). This required all levels of government to be held accountable for the health and wellbeing of Aboriginal and Torres Strait Islander peoples through the 'Closing the Gap' policy. Yet is this policy actually making any difference?

Utilising discourse analysis, based on the framework of philosopher Norman Fairclough (2003, 2010, 2015), an examination of the 'Closing the Gap' policy documents and subsequent performance indicator reports is being conducted. This research methodology allows the researcher to determine who is speaking within the policy, why they are speaking, who has allowed them to speak, whether they truly represent Aboriginal and Torres Strait Islander peoples, what historical influences may or may not exist, and how it all impacts on nursing as a health profession today.

As a result of undertaking this research, several publications have been produced to illuminate progress of government action and/or inaction. Advocating on behalf of Aboriginal and Torres Strait Islander peoples will continue to raise the profile of the inequities in health experienced within Australia. As a nurse, and having witnessed and experienced discrimination as a result of my cultural background, this research provides an opportunity for me to raise the profile of disadvantage to those who hold the power to make changes in social policy.

Key message for undergraduate health students: Regardless of your cultural background, everyone in our society has the right to be treated with respect, dignity and fairness. Nurses are a large professional group that can influence social change and lobby for changes in government policy within Australia and around the globe. Part of the nursing role is to advocate on behalf of our patients and even more so for marginalised groups. We have opportunities in our everyday practice to model behaviour that is culturally respectful and inclusive. As a professional group, nurses should be advocating, supporting and adding our voice to those who are disempowered, so that those who hold the power listen and make genuine changes to policy that eliminate discrimination and bias and improve the overall health and wellbeing of all within our diverse community.

Conclusion

In this chapter we have touched on the strengths of and understandings required to undertake Aboriginal and Torres Strait Islander research. Collaboration, consultation and reciprocity are key elements of building successful research partnerships. For research to be sustainable, all Australians should have some understanding of the strength of Aboriginal and Torres Strait Islander research and research methods.

SUMMARY

In this chapter we have explored concepts and terms that are relevant to Aboriginal and Torres Strait Islander research within the healthcare setting. This chapter has discussed and proved examples of a range of methods and complexities that are relevant to researchers. It has also highlighted the brilliant work of contemporary Aboriginal and Torres Strait Islander researchers within Australia.

Learning concept 1

Develop some understanding of Aboriginal and Torres Strait Islander health research: Historically, the majority of Indigenous research has been carried out by non-Indigenous people and has not been a positive experience for many Aboriginal and Torres Strait Islander communities. Researchers have a responsibility to cause no harm, but traditional forms of research have been a source of distress for Aboriginal and Torres Strait Islander peoples due to inappropriate methods and practices.

Learning concept 2

Explore ethical research principles relevant to Aboriginal and Torres Strait Islander health research: AIATSIS has 14 key principles that can be grouped under six broad categories: rights, respect and recognition; negotiation, consultation, agreement and mutual understanding; participation, collaboration and partnership; benefits, outcomes and giving back; managing research: use, storage and access; and reporting and compliance (see Table 4.1).

Learning concept 3

Identify the key aspects of Aboriginal and Torres Strait Islander research processes: The three key processes of Aboriginal and Torres Strait Islander research are community participation, lengthy process and engagement. There is an interrelationship between these processes and each element is dependent on the others.

Learning concept 4

<u>Explore Aboriginal and Torres Strait Islander research methodologies:</u> Indigenous methodology emerged from the Canadian and Native American communities, gaining momentum in Australia in the early 1990s. Fundamentally, Indigenous research methodology decolonises and incorporates an epistemological stance where Indigenous worldviews are the focus and drive the methodological framework.

Learning concept 5

<u>Explore examples of key Aboriginal and Torres Strait Islander research champions:</u> Four Aboriginal and Torres Strait Islander health research champions were showcased. Each case study revealed the researcher's nation, research area and clinical expertise, and provided advice for undergraduate health students considering research with Aboriginal and Torres Strait Islander communities.

REVISION QUESTIONS

1. What are your initial responses to this chapter?
2. What have you learnt about research and Aboriginal and Torres Strait Islander research methodologies?
3. Critique Aboriginal and Torres Strait Islander research methodologies. How have they been implemented in healthcare research?
4. How could yarning be used beyond research methods?
5. What is the importance of community participation?
6. What is your understanding of research ethics in relation to Aboriginal and Torres Strait Islander peoples?

FURTHER READINGS/ADDITIONAL RESOURCES

Aboriginal Health & Medical Research Council of NSW. (1998). *Aboriginal Health & Medical Research Council Ethics Committee*. Retrieved from http://www.ahmrc.org.au/ethics.html

Australian Institute of Aboriginal and Torres Strait Islander Studies (AIATSIS). (2016). *Research*. Retrieved from https://aiatsis.gov.au/research

REFERENCES

Atkinson, J. (2002). *Trauma trails: Recreating song lines*. North Melbourne: Spinifex Press.

Australian Institute of Aboriginal and Torres Strait Islander Studies. (2012). *Guidelines for ethical research in Australian Indigenous studies*. Retrieved from https://aiatsis.gov.au/sites/default/files/docs/research-and-guides/ethics/gerais.pdf

Baydala, L., Ruttan, L., & Starkes, J. (2015). Community-based participatory research with Aboriginal children and their communities: Research principles, practice and the social determinants of health. *First Peoples Child & Family Review, 10*(2), 82-94.

Bessarab, D., & Ng'andu, B. (2010). Yarning about yarning as a legitimate method in indigenous research. *International Journal of Critical Indigenous Studies, 3*(1), 37-50.

Cochran, P., Marshall C. A., Garcia-Downing, C., Kendall, E., Cook, D., McCubbin, L., & Gover, R. (2008). Indigenous ways of knowing: Implications for participatory research and community. *American Journal of Public Health, 1*(98), 22-27.

Council of Australian Governments. (2008). *National partnership agreement on closing the gap in Indigenous health outcomes.* Federal Financial Relations. Canberra: Australian Government.

Couzos, S., Nicholson, A., Hunt, M., Davey, M. E., May, J., Bennet, P. T., & Thomas, D. (2015). Talking about the Smokes: A large-scale, community-based participatory research project. *The Medical Journal of Australia, 202*(10), 13-19.

Fairclough, N. (2003). *Analysing discourse: Textual analysis for social research.* New York: Routledge.

Fairclough, N. (2010). *Critical discourse analysis: The critical study of language.* United Kingdom: Pearson Education.

Fairclough, N. (2015). *Language and power.* New York: Routledge.

Geia, L. K., Hayes, B., & Usher, K. (2013). Narrative or yarning/Aboriginal storytelling: Towards an understanding of an indigenous perspective and its implications for research practice. *Contemporary Nurse: A Journal for the Australian Nursing Profession, 46*(1), 13-17.

Greene, M. J. (2014). On the inside looking in: Methodological insights and challenges in conducting qualitative insider research. *The Qualitative Report, 19*(29), 1-13. Retrieved from https://nsuworks.nova.edu/tqr/vol19/iss29/3

Kemmis, S., McTaggart, R., & Nixon, R. (2014). Introducing critical participatory action research. *The Action Research Planner* (pp. 1-31). Singapore: Springer.

Kovach, M. (2009). *Indigenous methodologies: Characteristics, conversations, and contexts.* Toronto: University of Toronto Press.

Laycock, A., Walker, D., Harrison, N., & Brands, J. (2011). *Researching indigenous health: A practical guide for researchers.* Melbourne: The Lowitja Institute.

Martin, K. (2003). Ways of knowing, ways of being and ways of doing: A theoretical framework and methods for indigenous research and indigenist re-search. *Journal of Australian Studies, 76*, 203-217.

McMurray, A. (2003). *Community health and wellness: A socioecological approach.* Australia: Elsevier.

Moreton-Robinson, A. M. (2017). *National Indigenous Research and Knowledges Network (NIRAKN) annual report 2016.* Brisbane: Queensland University of Technology.

Nakata, M. (2007). 'The cultural interface', in S. Phillips, J. Phillips, S. Whatman & J. McLaughlin (Eds.), (Re)contesting indigenous knowledges and indigenous studies. *Australian Journal of Indigenous Education, 36*(suppl.), 7-14.

Rigney, L. (1997). Internationalisation of an Indigenous anti-colonial cultural critique of research methodologies: A guide to indigenist research methodology and its principles. *Journal for Native American Studies, 14*(12), 109-121.

Sherwood, J. (2010). *Do no harm: Decolonising Aboriginal health research.* (Doctoral dissertation). University of New South Wales, Sydney. Retrieved from http://healthbulletin.org.au/articles/do-no-harm-decolonising-aboriginal-health-research/

Smith, L. T. (1999). *Decolonizing methodologies: Research and Indigenous peoples.* Dunedin: University of Otago Press.

VicHealth Koori Health Research and Community Development Unit. (2001). Research—understanding ethics: Community report. Melbourne: VKHRCDU, University of Melbourne.

Voyle, J. A., & Simmons, D. (1999). Community development through partnership: Promoting health in an urban indigenous community in New Zealand. *Social Science and Medicine, 49*(8), 1035-1050.

West, R., Stewart, L., Foster, K., & Usher, K. (2012). Through a critical lens: Indigenist research and the Dadirri method. *Qualitative Health Research, 22*(11), 1582-1590.

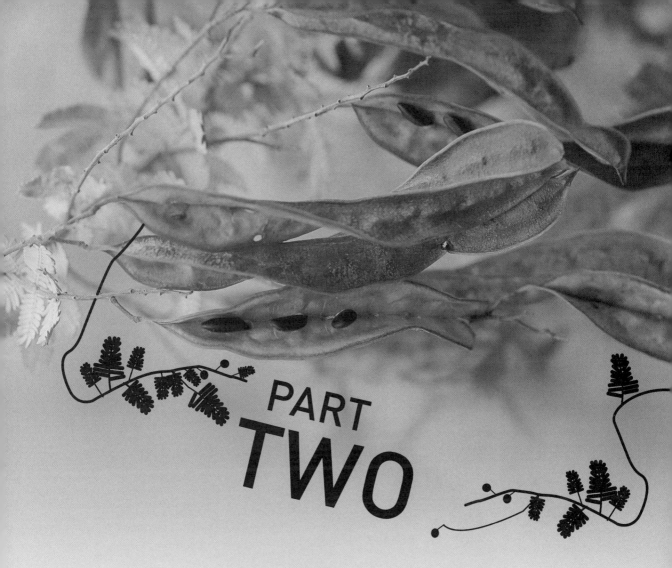

PART
TWO

Contexts of healthcare

This section will introduce key health systems that will enable your development and growth in Aboriginal and Torres Strait Islander peoples' healthcare. This section is important to consider in relation to the Australian National Health priorities and will provide practical advice and support when embarking on care.

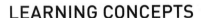

CHAPTER **FIVE**

Aboriginal and Torres Strait Islander peoples' cardiovascular health and wellness

Brett Biles, Megan Smith and Amali Hohol, with Darren Wighton

LEARNING CONCEPTS

Studying this chapter should enable you to:

1. identify the national prevalence of cardiovascular disease in Aboriginal and Torres Strait Islander communities.
2. identify the risk factors of cardiovascular disease in Aboriginal and Torres Strait Islander communities.
3. determine both the nurse and allied health professional's role in offering management options to Aboriginal and Torres Strait Islander people with cardiovascular disease.
4. describe how nurses and allied health professionals can promote positive health behaviours for Aboriginal and Torres Strait Islander people with cardiovascular disease, as well as the families and/or carers, to meet specific supportive care needs.
5. describe safe and culturally appropriate strategies for Aboriginal and Torres Strait Islander people with cardiovascular disease.

KEY TERMS

Aboriginal Community Controlled Health Service (ACCHS)
cardiovascular disease (CVD)
cardiac rehabilitation (CR)

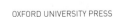

Introduction

This chapter will assist you to develop the skills and knowledge to use when providing care to an Aboriginal and Torres Strait Islander client with cardiovascular disease (CVD) or a client who is at risk of developing CVD.

Cardiovascular disease (CVD)

cardiovascular disease The term used to describe all conditions and diseases that affect the heart and blood vessels.

Cardiovascular disease (CVD) is the term used for all conditions and diseases that affect the heart and blood vessels (Baker Heart & Diabetes Institute, 2012). Coronary heart disease (ischaemic heart disease), cerebrovascular disease (stroke), hypertension and rheumatic heart disease are specific types of CVD (World Health Organization, 2016).

The life expectancy for Aboriginal and Torres Strait Islander people born between 2010 and 2012 has been estimated to be 69.1 years for males and 73.7 years for females, approximately 10 to 11 years less than the estimates for non-Indigenous males and females (Australian Indigenous HealthInfoNet, 2018). Aboriginal and Torres Strait Islander peoples experience higher rates of morbidity and mortality from chronic illness than non-Indigenous Australians. CVD was the leading cause of death in Aboriginal and Torres Strait Islander peoples from 2011 to 2015 and was responsible for 24% of all deaths (Australian Institute of Health and Welfare, 2016b). The leading cardiovascular conditions contributing to higher mortality rate are coronary heart disease, stroke and hypertensive disease (Australian Institute of Health and Welfare, 2016b). In 2012–16 in South Australia, Western Australia, Queensland, New South Wales and the Northern Territory, the death rate for Indigenous men and women in the 25–35 years age group was 13.5 times higher than non-Indigenous men and women; and in the age group of 35–44 years the death rate was 10 times higher than non-Indigenous men and women (see Figure 5.1).

The reasons for the poorer health outcomes of Aboriginal and Torres Strait Islander peoples compared to non-Indigenous people are complex, but represent a combination of factors including historical, social, cultural, economic, geographical and community factors (Australian Indigenous HealthInfoNet, 2013). These factors are discussed in detail in Chapter 6.

Risk factors of cardiovascular disease (CVD)

Factors contributing to CVD among Aboriginal and Torres Strait Islander peoples are complex; they reflect a combination of broad historical, socio-cultural and economic factors as well as cardiac-specific risk factors (Penm, 2008). Risk factors for CVD (except

Figure 5.1 Prevalence of people reporting cardiovascular disease as a long-term health condition, by Indigenous status and age group, Australia, 2012–13

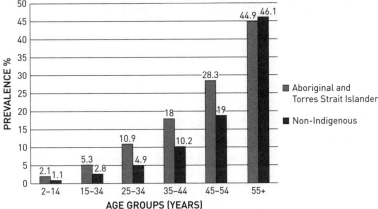

Source: Australian Indigenous HealthInfoNet (2018, p. 14).

rheumatic heart disease) can be split into two categories: behavioural and biomedical. Behavioural factors are based on the person's behaviour towards their health and include smoking, physical inactivity, poor nutrition and alcohol consumption. Behavioural factors can also be influenced by underlying social, economic, psychological and cultural factors. Bunker, Colquhoun and Esler (2003) have highlighted an important relationship between psychosocial factors and CVD, with social isolation, depression and a lack of social support having been highlighted as contributors to the development of CVD. Aboriginal and Torres Strait Islander peoples have been identified as an at-risk population whose social disadvantage is strongly associated with both psychosocial and modifiable risk factors, as identified by the National Heart Foundation of Australia (2010). Biomedical risk factors include hypertension, high blood cholesterol, obesity, diabetes and chronic kidney disease. These biomedical risk factors can be influenced by modifications to behaviour and lifestyle or the use of medical interventions.

Table 5.1 highlights modifiable (behavioural and biomedical) and non-modifiable risk parameters, as well as related conditions of CVD (Australian Institute of Health & Welfare, 2016b; National Heart Foundation of Australia, 2010).

Table 5.1 CVD risk factors and related conditions

Modifiable behavioural and biomedical risk parameters	Non-modifiable risk parameters	Related conditions
Smoking status Blood pressure Serum lipids Waist circumference and body mass index Nutrition Physical activity level Alcohol intake	Age and sex Family history of premature CVD Social history including cultural identity, ethnicity, socio-economic status and mental health	Diabetes Kidney function Family hypercholesterolaemia Evidence of atrial fibrillation

Aboriginal Community Controlled Health Services (ACCHSs)

As discussed in Chapter 2, Aboriginal and Torres Strait Islander peoples have experienced ongoing challenges to health and wellbeing, due to past policies and practices, racism, discrimination, and loss of language and identity (Dudgeon, Wright, Paradies, Garvey & Walker, 2014). There have been positive changes to health and wellbeing for Aboriginal peoples and this has been led by **Aboriginal Community Controlled Health Services (ACCHSs)**.

It is important to reinforce that Aboriginal and Torres Strait Islander peoples' health is holistic, encompassing mental health and physical, cultural and spiritual health. Land is central to wellbeing. This holistic concept does not merely refer to the 'whole body' but is also steeped in the harmonised interrelations that constitute cultural wellbeing. These interrelating factors can be categorised as largely spiritual, environmental, ideological, political, social, economic, mental and physical. Crucially, it must be understood that when the harmony of these interrelations is disrupted, Aboriginal ill-health will occur (Swan & Raphael, 1995, p. 13).

ACCHSs aim to deliver holistic, comprehensive and culturally appropriate healthcare to the community that controls it, through a locally elected Board of management or board of governance. In 1971, Redfern Aboriginal Medical Service (AMS) was the first ACCHS to be established, and there are now more than 140 ACCHSs in metropolitan, regional and remote areas of Australia. They range from large multi-disciplined services providing a wide variety of services, to small operations that rely on Aboriginal Health Workers and/or nurses to provide the bulk of primary-care services, with a preventive, health-education focus (National Aboriginal Community Controlled Health Organisation, 2018).

Aboriginal Community Controlled Health Service (ACCHS) A primary healthcare service initiated and operated by a local Aboriginal community to deliver holistic, comprehensive and culturally appropriate healthcare to the community that controls it.

Case study 5.1

Darren's story

Darren is a 49-year-old Aboriginal man who has been married for 23 years; he has two older teenage sons who still live at home. He lives in a regional city with good access to Aboriginal Health Services. Darren was diagnosed with type 2 diabetes when he was 34 years old and is insulin dependent (via daily injections). Darren has been managing his diabetes with fluctuating results since his initial diagnosis.

When Darren was 42 he developed chest pain and was admitted to Albury Base Hospital intensive care unit from his home. On presentation to the hospital Darren was assessed and then after three days of no pain was referred to a Melbourne hospital for follow-up due his family's history with CVD. In Melbourne Darren had an angiogram that confirmed that he had an acute non-ST elevated myocardial infarction as a result of one coronary artery blockage. Initial treatment included a percutaneous coronary intervention (PCI). Darren underwent the insertion of one stent to reopen his blocked coronary artery.

Darren spent one week in Melbourne following his PCI and was discharged home with follow-up care to be provided. Darren was referred to cardiac rehabilitation on his return home.

Darren attended cardiac rehabilitation at his local hospital for seven weeks. He enjoyed some but not all aspects of the program. He enjoyed the exercise and health literacy aspect of the program, but struggled with the unrealistic expectations of the healthy eating aspect. Darren felt a sense of isolation being the only Aboriginal person in the cardiac rehabilitation program.

CRITICAL REFLECTION QUESTIONS

- What are your initial thoughts and responses after reading this case study?
- Why do you think Darren felt a sense of isolation?
- Why is a family history of CVD an important factor when diagnosing CVD?

Providing culturally appropriate nursing care

As individuals we often only recognise another's culture when it differs from our own. It is, however, important to acknowledge that Australia is a culturally diverse nation, and as such, the demand for culturally competent nursing care is high (Baghdadi & Ismaile, 2018). The complexities associated with one's culture can result in misunderstandings, conflict, negative attitudes, discrimination and stereotyping between the client and nurse, thus negatively impacting the health and wellbeing of the client (Almutairi, Adlan & Nasim, 2017).

Nurses and midwives are the largest group of health professionals within the healthcare sector, with approximately 353,000 registered in 2014 (Australian Institute of Health and Welfare, 2016a). These statistics reflect that nurses and midwives account for three times the full-time equivalent of the next-largest health profession, that of medical practitioners. As nurses account for such a significant percentage of the healthcare workforce, it is imperative that cultural competence is embedded in the profession and therefore the provision of care.

In recent years, research has been undertaken that examines the significant impact cultural differences can have in terms of healthcare inequalities. Moreover, this research has explored the physical, spiritual, social and psychological manner in which diversity impacts the cultural safety of at risk populations (Almutairi, Adlan & Nasim, 2017). Within Australia, and in the context of caring for Aboriginal and Torres Strait Islander peoples, there are a number of cultural factors that nurses must consider when providing culturally competent care. Respect is fundamental, particularly in relation to acknowledging and understanding how historical events have impacted on Aboriginal and Torres Strait Islander peoples' health and wellbeing. This understanding must then be incorporated into the provision of care to ensure that it is culturally safe (West, Mills, Rowland & Creedy, 2018). Reflection and advocacy also must be considered. Reflection upon a nurse's own culture is necessary, and the nurse must critically reflect on how their professional cultural and social positioning may impact care provided to others with differing cultural values, norms and beliefs (West et al., 2018).

Culturally responsive communication is also important in terms of quality nursing practice. The nurse–client relationship is underpinned by effective communication. It is through the development of effective communication that trust is established between the care provider and the client. Yet, in the absence of culturally responsive and appropriate communication, the therapeutic relationship can be damaged, resulting in an inability to achieve nursing goals (Crawford, Candlin & Roger, 2017). Nurses must develop the ability to identify where potential misinterpretations may occur and implement strategies to avoid such occasions. The development of strong culturally appropriate communication skills will lead to higher levels of patient safety and patient satisfaction (Crawford, Candlin & Roger, 2017).

A nurse's cultural competence is influenced by their individual experiences of culture, either directly or indirectly. When a nurse experiences intercultural uncertainty—that is, a lack of knowledge and understanding of the attitudes and behaviours of those from a different cultural background—this can greatly impact their ability to provide safe, effective, culturally competent nursing care (Ahn, 2017). Nurses must make a conscious effort to reduce their intercultural uncertainty. Through the development of a deeper understanding of one's culture, nurses can better establish a rapport with their client, leading to better health outcomes (Ahn, 2017). See Chapter 1 for a discussion of the importance of Indigenous Australian cultural competence.

IMPLICATIONS FOR NURSING PRACTICE

Post-acute myocardial infarction

Acute coronary syndromes (ACS) are a subset of CVD and refer to angina and acute myocardial infarction (AMI). AMI can be further classified into ST-elevated myocardial infarction (STEMI) and non-ST elevated myocardial infarction (NSTEMI)

(Clune, Blackford & Murphy, 2012). The focus of this discussion will be on the nursing considerations of AMI. To achieve optimal patient outcomes, nurses must have the ability to recognise and manage the clinical presentation of an AMI. This includes being able to identify common clinical manifestations through rapid and accurate assessment processes and the implementation of evidence-based treatment interventions. The acute nursing management of an AMI will generally include comprehensive physical examination, diagnostic evaluation (including electrocardiogram (ECG), biomarker measurement and non-invasive imaging), initial and adjunctive drug therapy (outlined in Table 5.2), angiography with or without percutaneous coronary intervention (PCI), risk stratification, cardiac rhythm monitoring and general supportive measures.

Table 5.2 Initial drug therapy for acute myocardial infarction (AMI)

Intervention/treatment for AMI	Indications	Nursing considerations
Anticoagulants (unfractionated heparin, low molecular weight heparin, fondaparinux and bivalirudin)	Reduce thrombin-related events by inhibiting thrombin formation	Dependent on anticoagulant used
Aspirin	Inhibits platelet aggregation	Contraindicated in bleeding disorders, active peptic ulcer disease, hepatic disorders and aspirin allergy
Beta-blockers	Reduce myocardial oxygen demand by inhibiting heart rate, blood pressure and myocardial contractility	Contraindicated in vasospasm Avoid if heart rate <50 beats per minute
Morphine sulphate	Chest pain not relived by nitrates Anxiety	Monitor for hypotension and respiratory depression
Nitrates	Ongoing chest pain Cause venous and arterial dilation, reducing myocardial oxygen demand	Avoid if systolic blood pressure (SBP) <90mmHg
Oxygen therapy	Clinical significant hypoxemia Dyspnoea Reduces pain associated with myocardial ischemia	Maintain oxygen saturation >90%
Thrombolytic therapy	Reperfusion therapy is only indicated for STEMI Dissolves thrombi	Administration must occur within 3–4.5 hours of symptom onset Contraindicated in bleeding disorders, recent surgery trauma or other invasive procedure Monitor for bleeding and haemorrhage

Source: Cardiac Care Network (2013); Hamm, Bassand, Agewall, Bax, Boersma & Huber (2015).

Invasive angiography plays a key role in the management of AMI clients as it assists with confirming diagnosis and determining the appropriateness of coronary anatomy for PCI or coronary artery bypass grafts (Hamm, Bassand, Agewall, Bax, Boersma & Huber, 2015). PCI encompasses percutaneous transluminal coronary angiography (PTCA) and intracoronary stenting. The aim of these invasive procedures is to restore and/or improve the coronary blood flow to the affected myocardium (Olsen & Bowden, 2013). Despite PCI being associated with improved health outcomes, there is evidence indicating that Aboriginal and Torres Strait Islander peoples have lower rates of angiography and PCI. Walsh and Kangaharan (2017) explain that this is resultant from poor communication, language barriers, failure to include the client's family in healthcare conversations, lack of coordinated care and an absence of cultural safety within the healthcare setting.

General nursing care of the AMI client during the acute phase includes ongoing cardiac reassessment, including monitoring of vital signs. It is recommended that the client limits physical activity and remains on bed rest to reduce myocardial oxygen demand. The AMI client should have a pain-management plan in place to ensure episodes of cardiac chest pain are effectively managed. Repeat ECGs and pathology will also be required (Olsen & Bowden, 2013). Aboriginal and Torres Strait Islander clients have higher rates of discharge from hospital against medical advice. This issue is indicative of poor communication and inadequate cultural competence among healthcare providers, which leads to fear associated with hospitals. This issue in care provision highlights the importance of ensuring nurses and other healthcare providers clearly explain diagnoses and procedures to the client and their family; and, where possible, include Aboriginal health workers to facilitate a therapeutic decision-making process (Ilton, Walsh, Brown, Tideman, Zeitz & Wilson, 2014; Walsh & Kangaharan, 2017).

Post-AMI rehabilitation and education

Educating the AMI client should commence prior to returning to the community setting; that is, while the client is still within the acute care environment. Education should focus on prescribed medications, cardiac rehabilitation and risk modification (Cardiac Care Network, 2013). Effective long-term care post AMI must include management and reduction of risk factors, and this must be approached in partnership with the patient, their family and their community. For risk modification to be successful, there must be adequate patient education provided that allows the opportunity for the client to express their concerns and improve their understanding of their condition. Clients who assume an active role in their healthcare decisions have greater levels of adherence to treatment plans and are therefore more likely to engage in behaviours that improve their overall health and wellbeing (Trehearne, Fishman & Lin, 2014).

Cardiac rehabilitation (CR) is a fundamental component of post NSTEMI management, and therefore recommended for all ACS patients. CR is a long-term program that involves ongoing assessment, prescribed exercise, education, cardiovascular risk modification and psychosocial support. The primarily aim of CR is to minimise the physical and psychological impact of CVD, limit the risk of a secondary MI, control cardiac symptoms and increase quality of life (Cardiac Care Network, 2013). However, due to a range of barriers, Aboriginal and Torres Strait Islander people are often hesitant to engage with CR. In order to increase the uptake of this service, mainstream community health services must work alongside ACCHSs to ensure that the program acknowledges Aboriginal and Torres Strait Islander peoples' cultures and practices (National Heart Foundation of Australia, 2015).

cardiac rehabilitation (CR) A program where those with cardiac disease, their family and carers are supported by health professionals.

It is necessary to ensure that in the presence of complex comorbidities (for example, CVD and diabetes mellitus) long-term management focuses on the person, not the diseases in isolation. Clients such as Darren in this chapter's case study indicate a need for nurses to work in collaboration with other healthcare disciplines to ensure that the holistic needs of the client are addressed. Evidence indicates that clients who are provided with collaborative care management that focuses on addressing their complex comorbidities have great quality of life and higher levels of functioning (Trehearne, Fishman & Lin, 2014). For Aboriginal and Torres Strait Islander clients, the implementation of a local nurse cardiac care coordinator is linked to improved long-term care follow-up. The role of the care coordinator includes liaising with all members of the wider healthcare team and the client and their family. Continuity of care is also important. When the same nurse or other healthcare provider is used over a prolonged period of time, an enhanced therapeutic relationship can develop with Aboriginal and Torres Strait Islander clients (Walsh & Kangaharan, 2017).

Furthermore, encouraging patient involvement facilitates the provision of patient-centred care, whereby the individual client's needs, preferences and values in relation to their health are respected, acknowledged and integrated into the clinical decision-making process. This is particularly important in the context of an MI as research indicates that clients who are involved in decision making are less likely to have post-discharge cardiovascular complications than those who do not assume an active role in their own healthcare (Arnetz & Zhdanova, 2015).

Providing culturally and medically appropriate allied healthcare

A key element of the contemporary best practice management of cardiac disease is the inclusion of cardiac rehabilitation as part of a comprehensive care plan post an acute cardiac event. Attendance at cardiac rehabilitation is recommended in international guidelines as best practice in patients with heart disease (Dalal, Doherty & Taylor, 2015). The purpose of cardiac rehabilitation for individuals is twofold: to support secondary prevention by addressing modifiable risk factors for cardiac disease such as smoking cessation and dietary modification; and to support the development of optimal functioning post any cardiac event to enable full participation in employment and leisure activities (National Heart Foundation of Australia, 2015).

Individuals are typically referred to cardiac rehabilitation programs on presentation to a facility with a cardiac event or following an intervention. Allied health professionals play an important role in the conduct of cardiac rehabilitation. Allied health disciplines including physiotherapists, exercise physiologists, dietitians and occupational therapists are often involved due to the diet, exercise and lifestyle-modification components of cardiac rehabilitation.

In spite of the recognised benefits of cardiac rehabilitation, the inadequate implementation of secondary prevention activities such as cardiac rehabilitation has been recognised internationally (Piepoli et al., 2014). In Australia, participation rates for all Australians are comparable with the international experience, but are significantly worse for Aboriginal and Torres Strait Islander peoples. Evidence from the early 2000s states that Aboriginal people are under-represented in cardiac rehabilitation, with less than 5% of eligible participants attending (Shepherd, Battye & Chalmers, 2003). There is limited evidence to suggest that the attendance has significantly and systematically improved (Brown, 2010). A number of factors may impact the participation in cardiac rehabilitation and have implications for allied health practitioners during their interactions with Aboriginal and Torres Strait Islander people post a cardiac event.

Brown (2010) identified through a qualitative research study with Aboriginal and Torres Strait Islander people post acute coronary syndrome that the following areas influenced care outcomes:

- symptom recognition—the knowledge and interpretation of symptoms as representing a cardiac event
- seeking care—competing priorities for individuals related to family and other responsibilities, fear and mistrust, negative prior experiences, and family influence on seeking care
- delays to care—including delaying seeking help until symptoms were advanced and poor access due to socio-economic factors such as transport or phone access
- emergency management—extended wait times experienced when waiting for care
- in-hospital care—poor communication, lack of respect, feelings of invisibility, perceived racism, disengagement of family, clash of understanding, fear, and lack of a trusting relationship

- discharge—poor continuity, and little education and awareness about illness and treatment
- long-term management—being fixed, poor continuity, lack of access to rehabilitation, no outreach care and difficult navigation of the healthcare system.

IMPLICATIONS FOR ALLIED HEALTH PRACTICE

The role for allied health practitioners in the care of Aboriginal and Torres Strait Islander people post acute coronary artery disease will vary according to the professional's particular background and discipline-specific skills. For example, physiotherapists and exercise physiologists may be involved in exercise prescription to reduce risk factors and improve function, while dietitians will be involved in providing dietary advice. However, there are a number of generic implications for allied health based on the information in this chapter that are important during both the acute phase and the recovery phase.

During the acute phases, these implications include:

- ensuring that as a health professional you have undertaken training in cultural competency
- ensuring patients are referred to cardiac rehabilitation with a clear explanation—involving family—as to the need for cardiac rehabilitation and secondary prevention; important at this stage is clarifying that any procedure will not be a cure for life
- pursuing links on discharge to available programs and facilitating access. Where possible this would include selecting programs that are more culturally appropriate such as ones in community locations rather than hospitals. Where programs aren't available investigate innovative solutions.

Upon attendance at cardiac rehabilitation, implications include:

- ensuring cultural safety and respect, taking time to build relationships and engaging family
- ensuring a patient focus and addressing individual's particular challenges
- planning locations and activities that are relevant and supportive of Aboriginal and Torres Strait Islander peoples and their ability to access programs; for example, the design of programs such as that described earlier in this chapter by Dimer et al. (2013).

The key implication for allied health professionals is that attendance needs to be explicitly addressed and cannot be assumed to occur based on existing service models, especially where these have not been designed with cultural safety in mind.

This study by Brown looked at the whole care pathway, but many of these factors will specifically impact on the access to cardiac rehabilitation, including the lack of specific referral, the understanding of the role of cardiac rehabilitation and the availability of programs. In 2005, the National Health and Medical Research Council published guidelines for cardiac rehabilitation and secondary prevention for Aboriginal and Torres Strait Islander peoples, which was based on best evidence at the time. With the publication somewhat dated it may no longer represent best practice; however, the publication made a number of key points in relation to providing culturally appropriate care including understanding the barriers. These cultural factors included:

- 'Not enough black faces'—too few Aboriginal and Torres Strait Islander health professionals involved in providing cardiac rehab.
- Lack of communication and understanding of cultural factors that influence health behaviours—including a holistic view of health.
- Poor continuity of care—people falling between gaps in care between services (especially where this involves travelling long distances), weak links to Aboriginal Health Services and a lack of flexibility.
- Lack of community involvement and consultation in design—including a lack of utilising the leadership of Elders in the community.
- Location—such as hospitals that are not associated with recovery.

The National Heart Foundation of Australia (2015) produced guidelines designed to improve participation in cardiac rehabilitation for Aboriginal and Torres Strait Islander peoples; they recommended:

- providing culturally secure programs that use practices such as flexible appointments, culturally secure settings, engaging family members and improving relationships.
- ensuring effective referral systems, including clear communication between services and automatic referrals.
- implementing cardiac rehabilitation according to evidence-based guidelines so quality care is provided, particularly in settings other than traditional locations.
- providing cultural awareness training for allied health.
- ensuring service delivery options are considered where there are workforce gaps in allied healthcare, such as remote, rural and regional areas.
- developing dedicated and culturally appropriate resources.

There are some examples that support the idea that cardiac rehabilitation programs designed with cultural safety in mind can be effective in improving health outcomes for Aboriginal and Torres Strait Islander peoples. Dimer et al. (2013) reported on a cardiac rehabilitation program delivered through an Aboriginal Medical Service. These authors reported improved attendance and positive health outcomes. The model that was implemented was characterised by flexible attendance; a culturally sensitive location; community support and encouragement; holistic elements in the program, such as social determinants of health; yarning (discussed in Chapter 4); and responding to requests for information.

The National Heart Foundation of Australia has developed resources to guide and enable the explicit support of Aboriginal and Torres Strait Islander peoples in appropriate cardiac care. An example is the development of the quality-improvement toolkit, *Improving health outcomes for Aboriginal and Torres Strait Islander peoples with Acute Coronary Syndrome* (National Heart Foundation of Australia, n.d.). This toolkit is designed to support health professionals to meet standards of care related to clinical and cultural safety, and ultimately improve the quality of outcomes for Aboriginal and Torres Strait Islander peoples. Examples of resources such as this toolkit provide useful frameworks for allied health professionals.

IMPLICATIONS FOR NURSING AND ALLIED HEALTH PRACTICE

Reflecting on Darren's health data

Darren's case study provides a useful reflection on factors that positively influenced his experience, but also factors that could further enhance his health outcomes. Based on the evidence described earlier in the chapter, Darren is somewhat exceptional as an Aboriginal man in that he was successfully referred to a cardiac rehabilitation program in a regional location that was available and that he was able to attend. However, there were a number of factors that may have improved his experience of the program. These could have included:

- locating the program in a community location rather than at the hospital
- involving more Aboriginal people in the program, whether they were healthcare workers, members of the community or other people who had a similar condition
- ensuring the healthcare workers had adequate cultural training to understand the factors that would influence Darren's ability to implement the recommendations
- ensuring the healthcare workers understood the socio-economic factors that might have impacted on Darren
- ensuring his family and other community members were included so Darren would have support when the program finished
- reviewing the continuity and integration of services.

Case study 5.2

Darren's story continued

Darren has been receiving regular health reviews at his local Aboriginal Health Service (AHS) since his initial myocardial infarction (MI). He reports that his health and wellness has fluctuated over the seven years since his MI. Darren

(Continued)

says that for the first three to four years post MI his health and wellbeing were very stable and he was managing his modifiable behavioural and biomedical risk parameters very well. He was doing this through regular health reviews at his local AHS, seeing a dietitian regularly, and being involved in multiple exercise programs (with the Koori knockout weight loss challenge being a program he attended regularly). During this period, Darren's health was fairly stable, which allowed him to have a clear focus on his health and wellbeing. However, over the past three years Darren's health and wellbeing has been on a slow decline. Darren has put this gradual decline down to life getting in the way. The table below represents a snapshot of Darren's health and wellbeing at four and seven years post MI.

Table 5.3 Darren's health data

	Myocardial infarction (MI) presentation	Four years post MI	Seven years post MI
Weight	140 kg	100 kg	125 kg
Height	190 cm	190 cm	190 cm
Blood pressure	188/160 mmHg	130/90 mmHg	142/110 mmHg
Blood glucose level	14.5 mmol/L	6.2 mmol/L	12.5 mmol/L
Waist circumference	135 cm	110 cm	120 cm
Smoking status	Nil	Nil	Nil
Diet	Very poor: Large amounts of processed food Limited intake of fruit and vegetables Soft drink 2 × 1.25 L bottles per day	Fairly good: Regular intake of fruit and vegetables Minimal takeaway food Chicken, fish, red meat Minimal soft drink (diet Pepsi) 1–2 × 600 mL per week	Good to poor: Regular intake of fruit and vegetables Intermittent take-away food (twice per week) Biggest concern is portion sizes are still too large
Exercise	Very sedentary	Very active	Active to sedentary
Insulin dependent (via injections)	Yes	No	Yes

CRITICAL REFLECTION QUESTIONS

- After reviewing the snapshot of Darren's health and wellbeing, what key factors should you be focusing on with Darren, and why?
- Why is long-term management of cardiovascular disease so important for Darren?
- As one of the team members involved in Darren's case, develop a plan of care that considers his long-term needs and suggest preventative strategies that could be implemented to address these.

Conclusion

Cardiovascular disease is the leading cause of death for Aboriginal and Torres Strait Islander people. Nurses and allied health professionals are in an ideal position to improve health and wellbeing of Aboriginal and Torres Strait Islander people and the communities they live in by ensuring that access to health services and health promotion is delivered in a culturally safe environment that allows Aboriginal and Torres Strait Islander people to have and make informed decisions on their health and wellbeing.

SUMMARY

Throughout this chapter, you have explored the skills and knowledge required to utilise when providing care to an Aboriginal and Torres Strait Islander client who has CVD or is at risk of developing CVD.

Learning concept 1

Identify the national prevalence of cardiovascular disease in Aboriginal and Torres Strait Islander communities: Cardiovascular disease (CVD) is the leading cause of death in Aboriginal and Torres Strait Islander peoples. CVD was responsible for 24% of all deaths from 2011 to 2015.

Learning concept 2

Identify the risk factors of cardiovascular disease in Aboriginal and Torres Strait Islander communities: Risk factors for CVD (except rheumatic heart disease) can be split into two categories: behavioural and biomedical. Behavioural factors are based on the person's behaviour and include smoking, physical inactivity, poor nutrition and alcohol consumption. Biomedical risk factors such as hypertension, high blood cholesterol, obesity, diabetes and chronic kidney disease can be influenced by modifications to behaviour, lifestyle or the use of medical interventions.

Learning concept 3

Determine both the nurse and allied health professional's role in offering management options to Aboriginal and Torres Strait Islander people with cardiovascular disease: Management options need to be centred on the client and their individual needs, ranging from acute presentation to ongoing chronic disease management.

Learning concept 4

Describe how nurses and allied health professionals can promote positive health behaviours for Aboriginal and Torres Strait Islander people with cardiovascular disease, as well as the families and/or carers, to meet specific supportive care needs: Positive behaviours start with the health practitioner and their journey in cultural competence. Client advocacy, worldviews and beliefs all impact the care received and provided.

Learning concept 5

Describe safe and culturally appropriate strategies for Aboriginal and Torres Strait Islander people with cardiovascular disease: An ongoing journey of Indigenous Australian cultural competence is paramount. Refer to Chapter 1.

REVISION QUESTIONS

1. Why is culturally appropriate care important when dealing with Aboriginal and Torres Strait Islander peoples?
2. Why is it important to understand the relationship between the acute myocardial infarction and the long-term management of cardiovascular disease?
3. What are the common risk factors associated with the development of cardiovascular disease in Aboriginal and Torres Strait Islander peoples?
4. Review the case study of Darren. What are the health practitioner services that would be suitable to refer Darren to? Why did you choose these services?

FURTHER READINGS/ADDITIONAL RESOURCES

Australian Indigenous HealthInfoNet: https://healthinfonet.ecu.edu.au

National Aboriginal Community Controlled Health Organisation: https://www.naccho.org.au

REFERENCES

Ahn, J. W. (2017). Structural equation modeling of cultural competence of nurses caring for foreign patients. *Asian Nursing Research*, *11*(1), 65-73.

Almutairi, A. F., Adlan, A. A., & Nasim, M. (2017). Perceptions of the critical cultural competence of registered nurses in Canada. *BMC Nursing, 16*(1), 47.

Arnetz, J. E., & Zhdanova, L. (2015). Patient involvement climate: Views and behaviours among registered nurses in myocardial infarction care. *Journal of Clinical Nursing, 24*(3-4), 475-485.

Australian Indigenous HealthInfoNet. (2013). *Summary of Australian Indigenous health, 2012.* Perth: Australian Indigenous HealthInfoNet. Retrieved from http://www.healthinfonet.ecu.edu.au/overview

Australian Indigenous HealthInfoNet. (2018). *Overview of Aboriginal and Torres Strait Islander health status, 2017.* Perth: Australian Indigenous HealthInfoNet.

Australian Institute of Health and Welfare. (2016a). 2.3. Who is in the health workforce? *Australia's health 2016.* Retrieved from https://www.aihw.gov.au/getmedia/cce76972-bbfd-415c-9e9d-c68fac8243bd/ah16-2-3-who-is-in-the-health-workforce.pdf.aspx

Australian Institute of Health and Welfare. (2016b). *Australian burden of disease study: Impact and causes of illness and death in Aboriginal and Torres Strait Islander people 2011.* Canberra: Australian Institute of Health and Welfare.

Australian Institute of Health and Welfare. (2017). *Aboriginal and Torres Strait Islander health performance framework.* Retrieved 2018 from: https://www.aihw.gov.au/reports/indigenous-health-welfare/health-performance-framework/contents/summary

Baghdadi, N. A., & Ismaile, S. (2018). Cultural competency of nursing faculty teaching in baccalaureate nursing programs in the United States. *Australasian Medical Journal, 11*(2), 126-134.

Baker Heart & Diabetes Institute. (2012). *Cardiovascular disease.* Retrieved 2018 from: https://www.baker.edu.au/health-hub/fact-sheets/cardiovasculardisease

Brown, A. (2010). Acute coronary syndromes in Indigenous Australians: Opportunities for improving outcomes across the continuum of care. *Heart, Lung and Circulation, 19*(5-6), 325-336.

Bunker, S. J., Colquhoun, D. M., & Esler, M. D. (2003). Stress and coronary heart disease: Psychosocial risk factors. *Medical Journal of Australia, 178,* 272-276.

Cardiac Care Network. (2013). *Management of acute coronary syndromes.* Retrieved from https://www.corhealthontario.ca/ACS-management-in-remote-communities-FINAL-Sept-2013.pdf

Clune, S., Blackford, J., & Murphy, M. (2012). Management of the acute cardiac patient in the Australian rural setting: A 12-month retrospective study. *Australian Critical Care, 27*, 11-16.

Crawford, T., Candlin, S., & Roger, P. (2017). New perspectives on understanding cultural diversity in nurse–patient communication. *Collegian, 24*(1), 63-69.

Dalal, H., Doherty, P., Taylor, R. (2015). Cardiac rehabilitation. *BMJ, 351*, h5000. doi:10.1136/bmj.h5000

Dimer, L., Dowling, T., Jones, J., Cheetham, C., Thomas, T., Smith, J., McManus, A., & Maiorana, A. (2013). Build it and they will come: Outcomes from a successful cardiac rehabilitation program at an Aboriginal Medical Service. *Australian Health Review, 37*, 79-82.

Dudgeon, P., Wright, M., Paradies, Y., Garvey, D., & Walker, I. (Eds.). (2014). *Working together: Aboriginal & Torres Strait Islander Mental health and wellbeing principles and practice.* Canberra: Commonwealth of Australia.

Hamm, C. W., Bassand, J. P., Agewall, S., Bax, J., Boersma, E., & Huber, K. (2011). ESC guidelines for the management of acute coronary syndromes in patients presenting without persistent ST-segment elevation: The task force for the management of acute coronary syndromes (ACS) in patients presenting without persistent ST-segment elevation of the European Society of Cardiology (ESC). *European Heart Journal, 32*(23), 2999-3054.

Ilton, M. K., Walsh, W. F., Brown, A. D. H., Tideman, P. A., Zeitz, C. J., & Wilson, J. (2014). A framework for overcoming disparities in management of acute coronary syndromes in the Australian Aboriginal and Torres Strait Islander population. A consensus statement from the National Heart Foundation of Australia. *Medical Journal of Australia, 200*(11), 639-643.

National Aboriginal Community Controlled Health Organisation. (2018). *Introduction—The need for NACCHO.* Retrieved from https://www.naccho.org.au/about-nacho/naccho-history/

National Health and Medical Research Council. (2005). Strengthening cardiac rehabilitation and secondary prevention for Aboriginal and Torres Strait Islander peoples: A guide for health professionals. Canberra: NHMRC.

National Heart Foundation of Australia. (n.d.). *Improving health outcomes for Aboriginal and Torres Strait Islander peoples with acute coronary syndrome: A practical toolkit for quality improvement* (3rd ed.). Retrieved from https://www.heartfoundation.org.au/for-professionals/aboriginal-health/the-lighthouse-toolkit

National Heart Foundation of Australia. (2010). *Cardiovascular conditions.* Retrieved from https://www.heartfoundation.org.au/your-heart/cardiovascular-conditions/Pages/default.aspx

National Heart Foundation of Australia. (2015). Priority 6—*Improve participation in cardiac rehabilitation and ongoing care.* Retrieved from https://www.heartfoundation.org.au/images/uploads/main/Cardiac_rehab_INF-082-P_6__factsheet.pdf

Olsen, K., & Bowden, T. (2013). Nursing care of conditions related to the circulatory system. In A. M. Brady, C. McCabe & M. McCann (Eds.), *Fundamentals of medical-surgical nursing: A systems approach* (pp. 284-320). West Sussex: Wiley Blackwell.

Penm, E. (2008). *Cardiovascular disease and its associated risk factors in Aboriginal and Torres Strait Islander peoples, 2004–05.* Canberra: Australian Institute of Health and Welfare.

Piepoli, M. F., Corrà, U., Adamopoulos, S., Benzer, W., Bjarnason-Wehrens, B., Cupples, M., ... Giannuzzi, P. (2014). Secondary prevention in the clinical management of patients with cardiovascular diseases. Core components, standards and outcome measures for referral and delivery: A policy statement from the Cardiac Rehabilitation Section of the European Association for Cardiovascular Prevention & Rehabilitation. Endorsed by the Committee for Practice Guidelines of the European Society of Cardiology. *European Journal of Preventive Cardiology*, 21(6), 664-681. https://doi.org/10.1177/2047487312449597

Shepherd, F., Battye, K., & Chalmers, E. (2003). Improving access to cardiac rehabilitation for remote Indigenous clients. *Australian & New Zealand Journal of Public Health*, 27(6), 632-636.

Swan, P., & Raphael, B. (1995). *Ways forward: National consultancy report on Aboriginal and Torres Strait Islander mental health, part 1 and part 2*. Canberra: Australian Government Publishing Service.

Trehearne, B., Fishman, P., & Lin, E. B. (2014). Role of the nurse in chronic illness management: Making the medical home more effective. *Nursing Economic*, 32(4), 178-184.

Walsh, W. F., & Kangaharan, N. (2017). Cardiac care for Indigenous Australians: Practical considerations from a clinical perspective. *Medical Journal of Australia*, 207(1), 40-45.

West, R., Mills, K., Rowland, D., & Creedy, D. K. (2018). Validation of the first peoples cultural capability measurement tool with undergraduate health students: A descriptive cohort study. *Nurse Education Today*, 64, 166-171.

World Health Organization. (2016). *International statistical classification of diseases and related health problems, 10th revision*. Retrieved from http://apps.who.int/classifications/icd10/browse/2016/en#/XIX

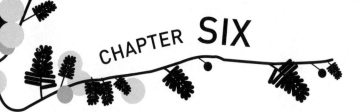

CHAPTER *SIX*

Aboriginal and Torres Strait Islander peoples' endocrinology health and wellness

Maryanne Podham, James Charles and Amanda Moses

LEARNING CONCEPTS

Studying this chapter should enable you to:

1. identify the national prevalence of endocrine disorders in Aboriginal and Torres Strait Islander communities.
2. identify the risk factors of endocrine disorders in Aboriginal and Torres Strait Islander communities.
3. discuss the role nurses and allied healthcare team members can play to provide management options, promote healthy behaviours and effectively communicate with Aboriginal and Torres Strait Islander people with an endocrine disorder using safe and culturally appropriate strategies.

KEY TERMS

allied health professionals
empowerment
endocrine disorder
health literacy
metabolic syndrome

Introduction

This chapter will assist you in developing skills and knowledge to use when providing care to Aboriginal and Torres Strait Islander people with an endocrine disorder.

Endocrine disorders

Endocrine disorders are those that involve altered levels of specific hormones within the body. These conditions can be both acute and chronic and can lead to life-limiting illnesses. Globally in 2010 the burden of endocrine disease was the ninth greatest cause of death, with type 2 diabetes being the most prevalent endocrine disorder attributed to these deaths (Horton, 2013). Obesity and type 2 diabetes are considered to be global challenges of the adult population, while the rise in the incidence globally of type 1 diabetes continues with more than 500,000 children and adolescents requiring insulin treatment worldwide in 2015 (Diabetes Australia, 2015). Through advances in treatment options, conditions affecting the thyroid have reduced; however, the incidence of newborn fatalities and illness continues to rise in developing countries due to the lack of iodine in the prenatal diet. There have been recent scientific suggestions made about the role of endocrine organ function (or lack of) in the development of illness in the older adult, including osteoporosis and dementia. Much research is being conducted into the interrelationships between endocrinology, obesity and metabolism (Horton, 2013).

endocrine disorder A condition affecting the body and its function due to alteration in the secretion of, or body response to, a hormone.

So, what exactly does the endocrine system do? Primarily this body system regulates metabolic processes of the body. It is also responsible for regulating the reproductive system, controlling the balance of extracellular fluids and electrolytes (including sodium and potassium), regulating blood glucose levels, and stimulating growth and development during childhood and adolescence (Farrell & Dempsey, 2014).

Given the rising incidence of diabetes and associated metabolic syndrome conditions in both Aboriginal and Torres Strait Islander and non-Indigenous populations, these conditions will be the predominant focus of this chapter.

What is an endocrine disorder?

The endocrine system involves a range of complex interactions and interrelationships within the body to maintain growth, reproduction and adaptive changes in the body. An endocrine disorder occurs when there is either an excessive or insufficient function of an endocrine organ, leading to altered levels of a specific hormone within the body's blood system. An endocrine disorder can also occur if there is a mismatch between receptor function and an intracellular response to a hormone-receptor complex. For example, in primary hyperthyroidism the release of thyroid hormone increases, leading to a decrease in the thyroid stimulating hormone (McCance, Huether, Brashers & Rote, 2015). The endocrine system is made up of a number of organs including the pituitary gland, thyroid, pancreas, adrenal glands, ovaries (female) and testes (male). Disorders of the endocrine system include diabetes insipidus (pituitary gland; not related to type 1 or 2 diabetes), Graves' disease and Hashimoto's disease (thyroid), diabetes mellitus (pancreas) and Cushing disease (adrenal cortex) (McCance et al., 2015).

What is diabetes?

Burrow and Ride (2016), suggest that diabetes is the world's fastest-growing chronic disease. Type 1 diabetes is predominantly related to children with a non-functioning pancreas and is not linked to modifiable factors (Dandona et al., 2005). Diabetes mellitus or type 2 diabetes is a disease process characterised by chronic hyperglycemia, with disturbances of carbohydrate, protein and fat metabolism as a result of the pancreas not producing sufficient insulin, or when the body cannot use the insulin effectively, which is also known as insulin resistance (Santoro & Christopher, 2018). The aetiology of type 2 diabetes is not clear, but it is strongly linked to lifestyle factors such as obesity, increased abdominal fat, physical inactivity, a high-fat diet and a familial history (Farrell & Dempsey, 2014).

What is metabolic syndrome?

metabolic syndrome
A cluster of risk factors that results in a person presenting with hyperlipidaemia, hypertension and type 2 diabetes simultaneously.

Metabolic syndrome is a cluster of risk factors that increase the risk of developing type 2 diabetes, cardiovascular disease and renal disease due to microvascular complications. The risk factors include abdominal obesity, insulin resistance, impaired fibrinolysis, dyslipidemia and hypertension (O'Neill & O'Driscoll, 2014).

Risk factors of endocrine disorders in Aboriginal and Torres Strait Islander peoples

The risk of developing an endocrine disorder can be influenced by many factors other than individual lifestyle factors. Historical, social, cultural, socio-economic, geographic and community factors also influence health.

Historical factors

Traditionally Aboriginal and Torres Strait Islander populations lived a hunter-gather lifestyle, with reliance on renewable food sources, familial and cultural practices and the maintenance of a spiritual connection to the land. Following the arrival of Europeans in 1788, adverse changes in both physical activity and nutritional practices led to changes in the metabolic functions within Aboriginal and Torres Strait Islander populations. The first recorded case of diabetes in an Indigenous person was in 1923 (Burrow & Ride, 2016).

Social and cultural factors

Socially and culturally, Aboriginal and Torres Strait Islander peoples have traditionally gathered to celebrate as a community, often with neighbouring tribes. These gatherings saw the participation in many physical activities including dance and ball games, as well as the sharing of news, stories and feasting on local produce, much of which was gathered during the celebration (Sebastian & Donelly, 2013).

In more modern times, Aboriginal and Torres Strait Islander peoples continued to gather for social and cultural activities, with sport playing a very important part. However, many contemporary cultural gatherings are now less related to activity, but with feasting remaining as an important part. Providing food for visitors is about reciprocity, giving and sharing, and this is part of many traditional Aboriginal and Torres Strait Islander peoples' cultures. Unfortunately, this feasting without activity has had an impact on weight gain and potential endocrine disorders (Charles, 2015).

Socio-economic factors

Issues such as limited and inadequate housing, and unemployment leading to lack of financial resources, frequently lead to reduced self-esteem and a reliance on behaviours that are health risks, such as excessive alcohol and tobacco consumption (Waterworth, Dimmock, Pescud, Braham & Rosenburg, 2016).

It is well documented that despite some improvements, education and literacy levels remain low in many Aboriginal and Torres Strait Islander communities, which in turn also affects both community and individuals' health literacy (discussed later in this chapter). The impact of reduced education and literacy levels on socio-economic status affects many aspects of an individual's possible health outcomes, as well as the awareness of when ill health is being experienced. Low levels of health literacy and the other previously mentioned issues can also lead to psychological stress when seeking healthcare, and this can be further affected by a lack of affordable transport options to attend healthcare services (Gunstone, 2013).

Geographical factors

Access to treatment for endocrine and other health conditions can be problematic for many Aboriginal and Torres Strait Islander communities, especially in rural and remote areas. Place of residence is considered an extremely important aspect of Aboriginal and Torres Strait Islander peoples' culture and health, but this can impact on the availability of healthcare services. Approximately 34% of all Aboriginal and Torres Strait Islander peoples live in cities and 22% live in inner regional centres, with 21% living in outer regional areas, compared to 71%, 18% and 9% respectively for non-Indigenous Australians (Rickwood, Telford, Parker, Tanti & McGorry, 2014). The greatest difference in residence between Aboriginal and Torres Strait Islander peoples and other Australians is in remote and very remote areas, with approximately seven times more Aboriginal and Torres Strait Islander people living in remote areas (Rickwood et al., 2014). Aboriginal and Torres Strait Islander people living in remote areas are twice as likely to have endocrine disorders such as diabetes, which is often a consequence of a lack of fresh fruit and vegetables (due to availability and cost), and a heavy or excessive intake of refined cereals, sugar and sodium (Brimblecombe, Ferguson, Liberato & O'Dea, 2013).

Community factors

The importance of kinship and family are significant to many aspects of life within Aboriginal and Torres Strait Islander communities, including health and wellbeing. These links offer physical and psychological support in times of illness (Waterworth et al., 2016).

Lifestyle factors

Metabolic syndrome is associated with an increased risk of development of type 2 diabetes. Diagnosis of metabolic syndrome is based on abdominal obesity (measured by waist circumference), elevated blood glucose levels, elevated serum cholesterol and hypertension (Craft & Gordon, 2015). As identified by Dunning (2013), the increasing incidence of type 2 diabetes among Aboriginal and Torres Strait Islander peoples has been significant over the past decade, and this has been attributed to environmental factors, lifestyle factors and the increasing prevalence of childhood obesity in this population. The prevalence of metabolic syndrome among Aboriginal and Torres Strait Islander peoples has been estimated at 33% to 50% (Stanley, Laugharne, Chapman & Balaratnasingam, 2016). A study conducted by McDermott, Li and Campbell (2010) followed Aboriginal and Torres Strait Islander participants who had been diagnosed with metabolic syndrome, but with no diagnosis of diabetes, for six years and demonstrated a 20% progression to type 2 diabetes. They suggest that identifying metabolic syndrome is a reliable predictor of progression to type 2 diabetes. The significance of metabolic syndrome is that, if addressed appropriately, prevention of progression to type 2 diabetes can be achieved (Craft & Gordon, 2016; McDermott et al., 2010).

Demographics of endocrine disorders in Aboriginal and Torres Strait Islander peoples

The Australian Institute of Health and Welfare (2015) suggests that the fatal burden of endocrine disorders for Aboriginal and Torres Strait Islander peoples is eight times the rate of this burden for those of a non-Indigenous background. Endocrine disorders (including diabetes) are within the top five causes of death (see Figure 6.1) for Aboriginal and Torres Strait Islander people over the age of 45.

In relation to diabetes (the commonest form of endocrine disorder in Aboriginal and Torres Strait Islander peoples), in 2012–13 Aboriginal and Torres Strait Islander people were four times more likely to develop type 2 diabetes, while the incidence of diabetes being diagnosed during adolescence (10–14 years) was 6.9 times higher than in non-Indigenous populations within Australia. Aboriginal and Torres Strait Islander women were twice as likely to develop gestational diabetes (a condition that occurs during pregnancy) than non-Indigenous women, and hospitalisation rates due to diabetes were four times higher for Aboriginal and Torres Strait Islander peoples (Burrow & Ride, 2016). During this time, diabetes was the second leading cause of death for Aboriginal and Torres Strait Islander peoples, particularly for the female population with rates increasing by 15.2% compared to 2.1% in non-Indigenous populations (Burrow & Ride, 2016).

Figure 6.1 Age-standardised years of life lost (YLL) per 1000 population in Australian non-Indigenous and Indigenous populations, 2010

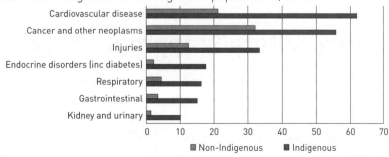

Source: Adapted from the Australian Institute of Health and Welfare (2015, Table 4.2).

Case study 6.1

Gerald's story

Gerald Hill is a 65-year-old Aboriginal male who lives by himself. He has two sons, who live with their families nearby. The city in which this family resides has good access to a broad range of Aboriginal medical services. Gerald worked as a carpenter until the age of 60, when he fractured his leg playing seniors' football. This led to a complicated recovery due to wound infection and a consequent delayed recovery and return to work. Added to this was the sudden and unexpected death of his wife, to whom he had been married for over 30 years. He gradually became less physical and socially active, which led to a weight gain and other associated symptoms. Gerald found it difficult to return to work, which led to him retiring early. Gerard attended the community health centre today for a check-up and the following information was identified:

- Weight: 110 kg
- Height: 185 cm
- Waist circumference: 105 cm
- Blood pressure: 164/93 mmHg
- Past history: hypocholesteremia and taking Atorvastatin 80 mg (maximum dose)

CRITICAL REFLECTION QUESTIONS

- What risk factors for endocrine conditions can you identify in the information provided on Gerard?
- What early intervention could be implemented to prevent Gerard from developing an ongoing condition in response to his current health status?

Providing culturally appropriate care

allied health professionals A range of healthcare providers—other than doctors, nurses and dentists—who work in multi-disciplinary teams to provide and support person-centred care.

Nurses and **allied health professionals** are in an ideal position to improve the health and wellbeing of Indigenous people, and in turn the wider community. However, to improve health outcomes, nurses also need to understand why there have been—and continue to be—disparities between the health and wellbeing of Aboriginal and Torres Strait Islander peoples and non-Indigenous Australians. Culturally appropriate care requires a nurse to understand the traditional practices and health beliefs of Aboriginal and Torres Strait Islander peoples, as well as the impact of historical injustices on the distrust towards the Western medical modes of healthcare (Hunt, Ramjan, McDonald, Koch, Baird & Salamonson, 2015).

Being able to understand the information provided in a healthcare setting is often taken for granted. When working with and providing healthcare to Aboriginal and Torres Strait Islander peoples, it is important to remember that there is not always comprehension of the language being used (Charles, 2017). English may be a second or third language in many tribal areas and there are still many Aboriginal and Torres Strait Islander people who do not speak or understand English very well. For many people this is a consequence of being denied the opportunity to learn English and receive an education (Hunt et al., 2015).

To enable changes to occur in the disparities of the health of Aboriginal and Torres Strait Islander peoples, healthcare services need to be patient-centred and not delivered from the perspective of the health professional. In the past, Aboriginal and Torres Strait Islander peoples have found themselves being examined, having a myriad of tests, receiving a diagnosis and being given treatment (for example, medication) without explanation or input, and without really understanding the need for or importance of the treatment (Charles, 2017). This lack of engagement and consultation is a likely reason why previous programs aimed at improving the health of these populations have not been successful.

To ensure culturally appropriate care is provided, there needs to be engagement and consultation that will empower the community. This will allow individual and collective input into what services are needed, how the services will be delivered, and how and when the community want them provided. This will lead to empowerment, genuine enthusiasm, and feelings of ownership of the service, which will increase community participation. The delivery of health services needs to be flexible and inclusive of the Aboriginal and Torres Strait Islander communities' perspectives and understanding of health and wellbeing, including remembering that all health professionals need to actively listen to the local community (Waterworth et al., 2016; Lambert, Luke, Downey, Crengle, Kelaher & Reid, 2014).

What is health literacy and empowerment?

Low levels of health literacy can lead to higher use of health services, reduced capacity to make informed healthcare decisions, and poorer health outcomes. Health literacy is considered a fundamental aspect of empowering healthcare users. The establishment of strong, focused, patient-centred partnerships between the user and the healthcare providers leads to a safer, inclusive health system that reduces inequities and disparity for all users (Australian Commission on Safety and Quality in Health Care, 2014).

How is health literacy defined?

health literacy Personal skills, knowledge, motivation and capacity to access, understand and use information to make decisions about one's own health and healthcare choices.

Health literacy needs to be viewed within two separate aspects: the health literacy of an individual, and the environment in which health literacy is being delivered. For an individual to improve their health literacy there needs to be a clear interplay between these two elements. The Australian Commission on Safety and Quality in Health Care suggests that health literacy involves a person's abilities and skills to find, analyse and adopt information to address their health needs. Further, the ability of the person to understand this information is dependent on how, where and when the information is presented, and on the relationship between the person giving and receiving the information (Australian Commission on Safety and Quality in Health Care, 2014). Vass, Mitchell and Dhurrkay (2011) suggest that for further improvements in the health literacy of Aboriginal and Torres Strait Islander peoples to occur, community and cultural literacy levels need to also be considered when planning and implementing healthcare. As mentioned previously, healthcare offered to many Aboriginal and Torres Strait Islander peoples has been based on biomedical theories with little to no consultation with the community or understanding of the cultural influences at play. For most Aboriginal and Torres Strait Islander peoples there is a strong interplay that links the causes of disease and illness with the land, law and relationships, which differs considerably to traditional biomedical models that have been imposed on them (Vass et al., 2011).

How do health literacy and empowerment interrelate?

empowerment The ability to take control of daily challenges without feeling overwhelmed.

Empowerment can be defined as the process of recognising and enhancing a person's ability to meet their needs, solve problems, locate the resources required to do so and to be in control of their life and wellbeing overall (Ayed & Aoud, 2017). Therefore, for there to be further improvements to the health and wellbeing of Aboriginal and Torres Strait Islander peoples, there needs to be increased involvement between the people, their environment, their culture and their needs. Information aimed at increasing knowledge and understanding related to endocrine issues such as diabetes needs to be provided in a manner that is understood by the various communities it is being offered in, with links between traditional medicine and the Western biomedical model clearly articulated (Vass et al., 2011).

What is health coaching and why is it important?

Health coaching is the use of skilful conversation to engage a patient in changing health behaviours in order to improve outcomes and prevent deterioration of a condition (Huffman, 2014). While health coaching embraces education, it is much more in-depth and considers the individual's situation and focuses on their identified needs and goals. With a focus on a holistic approach, health coaching uses a positive approach to health management, with the patient setting the agenda that will address their self-identified health concerns, which are determined through collaboration. The health professional is the coach, whose role it is to build a trusting relationship that promotes growth of motivational thinking and offers individualised treatment strategies and appropriate education to support the patient in developing goals that will be achievable and relevant to the issues that are causing them concern (Cinar, Freeman & Schou, 2018; Wolever, Dreusicke, Fikkan, Hawkins, Yeung, Wakefield & Skinner, 2010). Health coaching is considered to be a partnership between the health professional and the patient, and evidence is supporting improved outcomes when this technique is utilised, especially in the management of chronic disease (Huffman, 2014). Motivational interviewing is considered a crucial component of health coaching, and incorporates open-ended questions, empathy and empowerment through focused education, which supports behavioural changes and achievement of self-chosen goals (Wayne, Perez & Kaplan, 2015; Wolever et al., 2010).

Case study 6.2

Gerald's story continued

As information continues to be collected from Gerald, it is identified he has a medical history of asthma, which was previously well managed with a Salbutamol puffer. However, he is now finding that his breathlessness has worsened and has needed to add another medication, which he tells you is the 'purple puffer'.

Further to the information previously gathered, you have completed a thorough physical assessment and have noted the following.

	Last visit at 60 years of age	Findings at current visit/notes
Weight	65 kg	110 kg (increase of 45 kg in five years)
Height	185 cm	185 cm
Blood pressure	126/74 mmHg	164/93
Waist Circumference	80 cm	105 cm

(Continued)

Diet	Good intake of fresh fruit and vegetables, minimal take-away food, prefers food from home. Fish, chicken, lean red meat Minimal sugar intake Minimal alcohol Prefers water and tea No energy drinks or soft drink consumed	Reduced appetite for fresh fruit and vegetables, prefers foods that are quick to prepare (frozen meals) Daily use of alcohol (4–5 × 375 mL cans) Minimal water intake Increase in sugar, salt and processed foods Soft drink 2–3 × 1.25 mL bottles per day
Exercise	Very active	Very sedentary, due to injury and an increase in pain when walking, which reduces ability or desire to mobilise very far. Does not walk further than front gate; approx. 5 m
Smoking status	Nil	5–10 cigarettes per day, up to a packet a day on the weekend
Capillary blood glucose level	Random: 4.5 mmols	Random: 7.6 mmols
eGFR	89 mL/min	59 mL/min
Urinalysis	NAD identified	Mod glucose

Gerald reports that he has been voiding a lot over the last couple of weeks, is always thirsty, and always wants to eat. He has noticed a sore on his lower left leg that has been there for about a month and will not heal. He is treating it with Betadine and a dressing he got from the chemist (non-stick adhesive dressing).

Table 6.1 identifies the management considerations for the diabetic patient.

Table 6.1 Management considerations for the diabetic patient

Self-care behaviour	Considerations	Collaborate with
Diet	Review understanding of portion size, when to eat, what to eat and how often What are the healthiest choices? (Especially consider limited availability and access to food choices) Include family members in this discussion and planning	Dietitian Nutritionist Aboriginal Health Worker

Self-care behaviour	Considerations	Collaborate with
Activity	Discuss weight management options Discuss options of free activity close to home Discuss the role of activity in addressing lipid levels, blood pressure and stress	Physiotherapist Exercise physiologist Occupational therapist
Self-monitoring	Discuss self-monitoring of blood glucose	Community nurse Aboriginal Health Worker Diabetic educator Pharmacist/local chemist General Practitioner (GP)
Medication compliance	Discuss the importance of taking medications as directed Discuss possible side effects, interactions and sick day plans	Pharmacist GP Community nurse Aboriginal Health Worker
Risk-reduction considerations	Discuss use of alcohol, tobacco and illicit substances Discuss need for regular screening and check-ups for other diabetes-related conditions, including neuropathy and retinopathy Discuss how reduction of risk can enhance quality of life	GP Pharmacist Community nurse Aboriginal Health Worker Podiatrist Renal specialist Ophthalmologist Optometrist Cardiologist
Problem-solving skills	Develop a 'sick day plan' involving both the patient and the family Develop a plan that addresses progressive changes due to diabetes, the ageing process and end-of-life planning and choices Develop 'what if' plans Develop skills that enhance motivation, adherence and acceptance of the need to change one's lifestyle	Social worker GP Community nurse

Source: Adapted from Rice, Kocurek and Snead (2010).

IMPLICATIONS FOR NURSING PRACTICE

As is identified in Table 6.1, the role of the nurse in caring for Gerald (and other Aboriginal and Torres Strait Islander people with an endocrine condition) is multi-faceted and includes being the conduit between the patient and other healthcare team members. The Australian Health Ministers' Advisory Council (2017) suggests that the nurse's role should include patient-centred health promotion, focusing on a range of social and environmental strategies, in order for both the patient and the communities they live in to increase control over their health. Further responsibility lies in ensuring strong cooperative partnerships are developed between healthcare providers, including nurses, and the communities that interact with these services. Finally, an integrated approach to the detection and management options of an endocrine condition such as diabetes would be required. This would involve the nurse providing current diabetic education in a manner that was understood by the patient, including: medication administration and dose information; management of signs and symptoms of adverse conditions that can occur due to diabetes, including hypoglycaemic episodes, blood glucose management and recording of results; lifestyle choices (for example, alcohol use, diet, exercise and stress management); problem solving; and encouragement of self-management (Segal, Leach, May & Turnbull, 2013).

The diabetes educator is a role conducted by a suitably qualified health professional. This role involves a wide scope of practice, and in many Aboriginal and Torres Strait Islander communities the Aboriginal Health Worker may also undertake this role. Not only are these roles involved in the delivery of medication related information, but they are also fundamental in ensuring that a patient (such as Gerald) understands diabetes, why it has occurred and how it can be managed (King, Nancarrow, Grace & Borthwick, 2017).

CRITICAL REFLECTION QUESTIONS

- What are the factors to be aware of when assessing a patient for the development of diabetes mellitus?
- What is the significance of the symptoms of excess thirst, hunger and urination that Gerald is reporting?
- What other symptoms is Gerald presenting with that may be an indication of the development of diabetes mellitus?
- Develop a plan of care as the nurse or Aboriginal Health Worker with consideration of Gerald's immediate needs.

IMPLICATIONS FOR ALLIED HEALTH PRACTICE

From an allied health perspective, Gerald would need a multi-disciplinary approach to address his actual and potential health issues. Diabetes is the leading cause of adult blindness, kidney failure and cardiac disease (Rice, Kocurek & Snead, 2010). Diabetes is also the cause of the increased prevalence of lower extremity amputation in the Aboriginal and Torres Strait Islander population, compared to the non-Indigenous population, due to diabetic neuropathy (Schoen & Norman, 2014).

When working with a collaborative group, such as the allied health team identified in Table 6.1, it is important to ensure that the focus is on the patient and their needs, rather than the needs of the healthcare provider, which leads to a co-creation of knowledge in preference to simply the provision of information (Rice et al., 2010; Castro, Regenmortel, Vanhaecht & Sermus, 2016).

Regardless of the health team member involved in the treatment of the Indigenous patient, the development of an individual treatment plan using a step-by-step approach is helpful. The focus should be on identifying current behaviour and problem solving together. Family and community are important to Aboriginal and Torres Strait Islander peoples, and to increase motivation and adherence, these influences need to also be considered (Lambert et al., 2014).

Allied healthcare team involvement for Gerald

As mentioned previously, the incidence of diabetic foot ulceration and amputation is significantly higher in Aboriginal and Torres Strait Islander peoples than in the general population (Clement, 2011). To address this, a podiatrist would be involved to conduct a diabetic foot assessment, including nerve function test with monofilament and tuning fork, also testing vascular supply to the foot (Charles, 2017). An occupational therapist could conduct a home visit to assess Gerald's home, reviewing inside and out for falls risks, and the need for railings or other safety features to assist Gerald to be safe and maintain his independence (Roberts & Robinson, 2014). A dietitian would assist Gerald to review his food likes and dislikes and suggest ways for Gerald to make better choices when they are limited, such as at a sporting event (McArdle, Greenfield, Avery, Adams & Gill, 2017).

CRITICAL REFLECTION QUESTIONS

- How could a diagnosis of diabetes affect Gerald and his interactions with his community?
- Why would it be important for Gerald to be encouraged to self-manage his diabetes?
- What other services or strategies could allied health team members offer Gerald in relation to his diabetes?
- As one of the team members involved in Gerald's case, develop a plan of care considering his long term needs and suggest preventative strategies that could be implemented to address these.

Conclusion

Endocrine conditions, in particular diabetes, continue to contribute to the burden of illness for Aboriginal and Torres Strait Islander peoples of Australia. Nurses and allied healthcare workers are in the ideal position to improve the health and wellbeing of these people and the communities in which they live. It is vital that health promotion and education be delivered in a manner that is considerate of the needs of these patients and include traditional culturally appropriate care with less emphasis on biomedical models.

SUMMARY

This chapter has introduced the complexities associated with Aboriginal and Torres Strait Islander peoples' endocrinological health and wellness. When considering the burden of endocrine diseases in Aboriginal and Torres Strait Islander peoples through the key learning concepts, the role of health promotion and education is vital for nurses and allied health professionals.

Learning concept 1

Identify the national prevalence of endocrine disorders in Aboriginal and Torres Strait Islander communities: There is a high prevalence of endocrine disorders in Aboriginal and Torres Strait Islander communities, particularly type 2 diabetes, which is reported to be the second leading cause of death among Aboriginal and Torres Strait Islander peoples.

Learning concept 2

Identify the risk factors of endocrine disorders in Aboriginal and Torres Strait Islander communities: The development of an endocrine disorder in Aboriginal and Torres Strait Islander peoples is linked to a number of factors, including changes to the traditional hunter-gatherer lifestyle; sociocultural meetings that involve feasting; socio-economic limitations that lead to behaviours that are potentially a risk to health and access to services; and inadequate diet due to geographical isolation.

Learning concepts 3, 4, 5 and 6

Discuss the role nurses and allied healthcare team members can play to provide management options, promote healthy behaviours, and effectively communicate with Aboriginal and Torres Strait Islander people with an endocrine disorder using safe and culturally appropriate strategies: To ensure motivation, adherence and acceptance of the need for lifestyle changes, both Aboriginal and Torres Strait Islander patients and their community need to be involved in the planning, implementation and evaluation stages of healthcare. When addressing health literacy, consideration of traditional and cultural underpinnings of the causes of disease and illness need to be considered alongside the biomedical systems that are providing the healthcare to a patient. Nurses and allied healthcare team members are ideally placed to ensure this occurs.

REVISION QUESTIONS

1. Why is knowing the level of a patient's health literacy important when developing health education activities?
2. Why is it important to empower people in regards to managing their conditions?
3. What role does health coaching play in the support of a patient's acceptance of their condition?
4. Why is culturally appropriate care important when dealing with Aboriginal and Torres Strait Islander peoples?
5. Why is it important to understand the interrelation of diabetes and the metabolic syndrome?
6. What are the risk factors associated with the development of endocrine disorders in Aboriginal and Torres Strait Islander peoples?
7. Review the case study of Gerald and identify the three allied healthcare team members that would be suitable to refer Gerald to. Why did you choose these services?

FURTHER READINGS/ADDITIONAL RESOURCES

Australian Indigenous Health Information Network: https://healthinfonet.ecu.edu.au
Endocrine Society of Australia: https://www.endocrinesociety.org.au

REFERENCES

Australian Commission on Safety and Quality in Health Care. (2014). *Health literacy: Taking action to improve safety and quality*. Canberra. Retrieved from https://www.safetyandquality.gov.au/wp-content/uploads/2014/08/Health-Literacy-Taking-action-to-improve-safety-and-quality.pdf

Australian Health Ministers' Advisory Council. (2017). *National strategic framework for chronic conditions*. Canberra: Australian Government.

Australian Institute of Health and Welfare. (2015). *Australian burden of disease: Fatal burden of disease in Aboriginal and Torres Strait Islander people 2010.* Australian Burden of Disease Study Series No.2. Canberra: AIHW.

Ayed, M. B., & Aoud, N. E. (2017). The patient empowerment: A promising concept in healthcare marketing. *International Journal of Healthcare Management, 10*(1), 42-48.

Brimblecombe, J. K., Ferguson, M. M., Liberato, S. C., & O'Dea, K. (2013). Characteristics of the community-level diet of Aboriginal people in remote northern Australia. *Medical Journal of Australia, 198*(7), 380-384.

Burrow, S., & Ride, K. (2016). Review of diabetes among Aboriginal and Torres Strait Islander people. *Australian Indigenous HealthInfoNet.* Retrieved from https://healthinfonet.ecu.edu.au/healthinfonet/getContent.php?linkid=590810&title=Review+of+diabetes+among+Aboriginal+and+Torres+Strait+Islander+people

Castro, E. M., Regenmortel, T. V., Vanhaecht, K., & Sermus, W. (2016). Patient empowerment, patient participation and patient-centeredness in hospital care: A concept analysis based on a literature review. *Patient Education and Counselling, 99*, 1923-1939.

Charles, J. (2015). An evaluation and comprehensive guide to successful Aboriginal health promotion. *Australian Indigenous Health Bulletin, 16*(1), 1-7.

Charles, J. (2017). The Aboriginal Multiple Injury Questionnaire (AMIQ): The development of a musculoskeletal injury questionnaire for an Australian Aboriginal population. *Australian Indigenous Health Bulletin, 17*(3), 1-7.

Cinar, A. B., Freeman, R., & Schou, L. (2018). A new complementary approach for oral health and diabetes management health coaching. *International Dental Journal, 68*(1), 54-64.

Clement, Z. (2011). Diabetic foot ulcer management: Clinical and cost effectiveness of vacuum assisted closure therapy. *Aboriginal & Islander Health Worker Journal, 35*(2), 5-8.

Craft, J., & Gordon, C. (2015). *Understanding pathophysiology* (2nd ed.). Chatswood: Mosby Elsevier.

Dunning, T. (2013). Concepts of endocrine disorders. In S. Bullock & M. Hales (Eds.), *Principles of pathophysiology.* Frenchs Forrest: Pearson.

Farrell, M., & Dempsey, J. (2014). *Smeltzer & Bare's textbook of medical–surgical nursing* (3rd ed.). Sydney: Lippincott Williams & Wilkins.

Gunstone, A. (2013). Indigenous education 1991–2000: Documents, outcomes and governments. *Australian Journal of Indigenous Education, 41*(2), 75-84.

Horton, R. (2013). Endocrine disorders: Turning towards the road less travelled. *The Lancet & Endocrinology, 1*(1), 1. https://doi.org/10.1016/S2213-8587(13)70096-2

Huffman, M. (2014). Using motivational interviewing through evidenced-based health coaching. *Home Healthcare Now, 32*(9), 543-548.

Hunt, L., Ramjan, L., McDonald, G., Koch, J., Baird, D., & Salamonson, Y. (2015). Nursing student's perspectives of the health and healthcare issues of Australian Indigenous people. *Nurse Education Today, 35*, 461-467.

King, O., Nancarrow, S., Grace, S., & Borthwick, A. (2017). Diabetes educator role boundaries in Australia: A documentary analysis. *Journal of Foot and Ankle Research, 10*(28), 1-11.

Lambert, M., Luke, J., Downey, B., Crengle, S., Kelaher, M., & Reid, S. (2014). Health literacy: Health professional's understandings and their perceptions of barriers that Indigenous patients encounter. *BMC Health Services Research, 14*, 614-623.

McArdle, P. D., Greenfield, S. M., Avery, A., Adams, G. G., & Gill, P. S. (2017). Dietitians' practice in giving carbohydrate advice in the management of type 2 diabetes: A mixed method study. *Journal of Human Nutrition & Dietetics*, *30*(7), 385-393.

McCance, K. L., Huether, S. E., Brashers, V. L., & Rote, N. S. (2015). *Pathophysiology: The biologic basis for disease in adults and children* (7th ed.) Canada: Mosby Elsevier.

McDermott, R., Li, M., & Campbell, S. (2010). Incidence of type 2 diabetes in two Indigenous Australian populations: A 6-year follow-up study. *Medical Journal of Australia*, *192*(10), 562-565.

O'Neill, S., & O'Driscoll, L. (2015). Metabolic syndrome: A closer look at the growing epidemic and its associated pathologies. *International Association for the Study of Obesity*, *16*, 1-12.

Rice, D., Kocurek, B., & Snead, C. A. (2010). Chronic disease management for diabetes: Baylor health care systems' coordinated efforts and the opening of Diabetes Health and Wellness Institute. *Baylor University Medical Centre Proceedings*, *23*(3), 230-234.

Rickwood, D. J., Telford, N. R., Parker, A. G., Tanti, C. J., & McGorry, P. D. (2014). Headspace—Australia's innovation in youth mental health: Who are the clients and why are they presenting? *Medical Journal of Australia*, *200*(2), 1-4.

Roberts, P.S., & Robinson, M. R. (2014). Health policy perspectives: Occupational therapy's role in preventing acute readmissions. *American Journal of Occupational Therapy*, *68*, 254-259.

Santoro, N., & Christopher, D. (2018). Type 2 diabetes in the non-pregnant patient. An update on management options. *Contemporary OB/Gyn*, *63*(12), 29-48.

Schoen, D. E., & Norman, P. E. (2014). Diabetic foot disease in Indigenous people. *Diabetes Management*, *4*(6), 489-500.

Sebastian, T., & Donelly, M. (2013). Policy influence affecting the food practices of Indigenous Australians since colonisation. *Aboriginal Australian Studies*, *2*, 59-75.

Segal, L., Leach, M. J., May, E., & Turnbull, C. (2013). Regional primary care team to deliver best–practice diabetes care. *Diabetes Care*, *36*, 1898-1907.

Stanley, S. H., Laugharne, J. D. E., Chapman, M., & Balaratnasingam, S. (2015). Kimberley Indigenous mental health: An examination of metabolic syndrome risk factors. *Australian Journal of Rural Health*, *24*(5), 300-305.

Vass, A., Mitchell, A., & Dhurrkay, Y. (2011). Health literacy and Australian Indigenous peoples: An analysis of the role of language and worldview. *Health Promotion Journal of Australia*, *22*, 33-37.

Waterworth, P., Dimmock, J., Pescud, M., Braham, R., & Rosenburg, M. (2016). Factors affecting Indigenous West Australians' health behaviour: Indigenous perspectives. *Qualitative Health Research*, *26*(1), 55-68.

Wayne, N., Perez, D. F., & Kaplan, D. M. (2015). Health coaching reduces HbA1c in type 2 diabetic patients from a lower socio-economic status community: A randomised controlled trial. *Journal of Medical Internet Research*, *17*(10), 3-5.

Wolever, R., Dreusicke, M. M., Fikkan, J. J., Hawkins, T. V., Yeung, S., Wakefield, J., & Skinner, E. (2010). Integrative health coaching for patients with type 2 diabetes: A randomised clinical trial. *Diabetes Educator*, *36*(4), 629-639.

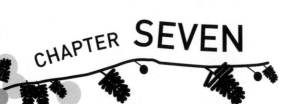

CHAPTER SEVEN

The early years

Ailsa Munns and Kristy Robson

LEARNING CONCEPTS

Studying this chapter should enable you to:

1. explore concepts of Aboriginal and Torres Strait Islander peoples' maternal and child health and wellbeing.
2. identify the importance of Indigenous Australian cultural competence for maternal and child health.
3. identify and explore social determinants of health impacting on Aboriginal and Torres Strait Islander peoples' perinatal health and the early years.
4. identify and explore interprofessional skills for working in culturally competent partnership with Aboriginal and Torres Strait Islander individuals, families and communities in the perinatal period and early years.
5. identify and explore the roles of nurses and allied health professionals working with Aboriginal and Torres Strait Islander families with young children.

KEY TERMS

interprofessional collaboration
perinatal period
primary healthcare
social determinants of health

OXFORD UNIVERSITY PRESS

Introduction

Throughout this chapter you will be asked to reflect on and consider the impacts of **social determinants of health**, culture and Indigenous Australian cultural competence (see Chapter 1) on the psychosocial health and wellbeing of Aboriginal and Torres Strait Islander women, their families, children and their communities during the preconception and perinatal periods and the early years of children's lives. As a registered nurse or allied health practitioner, you will need to reflect on your previous readings on cultural competence, and consider how these competencies translate into clinical practice in this important area and the implications for your professional competencies.

Addressing social determinants of health is enhanced by taking into account client strengths, a **primary healthcare** approach and interprofessional practice, all of which underpin culturally competent practice. This chapter will require you to explore concepts of Aboriginal and Torres Strait Islander peoples' maternal and child health and wellbeing and encourage critical reflection on how strengths-based, cultural competencies can be developed and applied to clinical practice.

First, it is important to review the national standards for Australian nursing and midwifery practice at http://www.nursingmidwiferyboard.gov.au/Codes-Guidelines-Statements/Professional-standards.aspx. These will help to guide you in your reflections and development of care for Aboriginal and Torres Strait Islander women, their families, children and their communities.

> **social determinants of health** Interrelated social factors that determine health and wellbeing.

> **primary healthcare** A philosophy of care based on social justice and an organising framework guiding health professionals to facilitate equitable social environments, equal access to healthcare and empowerment through public participation (McMurray & Clendon, 2015).

Health and wellbeing in the early years

Maintaining healthy growth and development for children in the early years is a multi-layered issue, with factors such as maternal perinatal health, family and community environments and social determinants of health impacting on their health and wellbeing. It is important to understand that Aboriginal and Torres Strait Islander peoples' holistic view of health can impact on their parenting practices. Physical, cultural, spiritual and social wellbeing are central to Aboriginal and Torres Strait Islander peoples' health (Australian Institute of Health and Welfare & Australian Institute of Family Studies, 2013), which is highlighted in Figure 7.1 and the definition from the 1989 National Health strategy: 'Health is not just the physical wellbeing of the individual, but the social, emotional and cultural well-being of the whole community. This is a whole of life view and it also includes the cycle of life-death-life' (National Aboriginal Health Strategy Working Party, 1989).

It can be seen that supporting parents in their role through individual, family and community engagement needs to encompass psychosocial strategies in order to maintain or improve the health and wellbeing of their children. Aboriginal and Torres

Figure 7.1 Interrelationships of holistic health

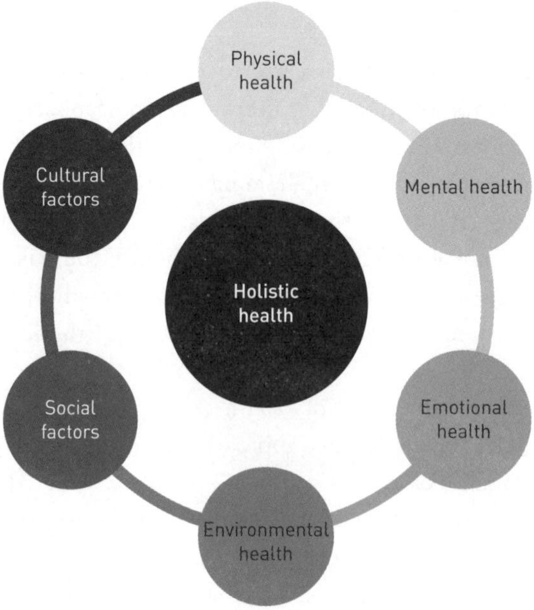

Source: Hampton and Toombs (2013, p. 76).

Strait Islander peoples are also linked to a predetermined system of kinship that can strongly affect their parenting interactions, relationships and responsibilities. Roles of family members will differ between regions and communities, so it is important to recognise these within each local area (Taylor & Guerin, 2014).

Social determinants of health are structures and conditions impacting on people's physical, social and emotional health and wellbeing. These interconnecting determinants relate to issues such as poverty, unemployment, lack of housing and social disadvantage. For Aboriginal and Torres Strait Islander families, these may be compounded by factors such as racism, cultural dislocation, dispossession and child removals, all of which pose risks of adverse developmental outcomes from pre-conception and conception through to the early years and adulthood (Zubrick, Shepherd, Dudgeon, Gee, Paradies, Scrine & Walker, 2014). The impact of poverty is noted to have a wide scope of adverse child health outcomes, including poor cognitive development and lower educational attainment in addition to less resources being available to parents, thereby reducing their chances to help their children (Emerson, Fox & Smith, 2015). However, there are distinctive characteristics of Aboriginal and Torres Strait Islander peoples' cultures that help to support parents in maintaining healthy development for their children, both in pregnancy and in the early years. In turn, these help to develop positive lifelong health trajectories. Feelings of connection to land, spirituality, kinship networks and cultural continuity are recognised as health protecting factors for children, parents and whole communities (Zubrick et al., 2014).

The unique health challenges faced by Aboriginal and Torres Strait Islander families are optimally addressed by strengths-based approaches to nursing and allied health practice. Opportunities to embrace strategies that protect and enhance health and wellbeing need to be recognised and incorporated into culturally safe practice approaches. These encourage working in partnership with parents, children and their communities to include their expertise within their own care, which, in turn, facilitates their empowerment, feelings of value, self-worth and respect. The ability of strengths-based approaches to enhance innovative, interprofessional practice in the early years has also been recognised (Fenton, Walsh, Wong & Cumming, 2015), with increasing recognition of significantly greater benefits for individuals and families experiencing complex physical and psychosocial needs (Schultz, Walker, Bessarab, McMillan, Macleod & Marriott, 2014). Community-based health professionals are well placed to use these courses of action in their practice settings to develop positive, enabling early life experiences rather than highlighting only deficits within people's personal and community environments.

Primary healthcare guides nurses and allied health professionals to assist people to develop equitable and socially just health settings. The principles of primary healthcare incorporate a guiding framework for care, incorporating the principles of accessibility to healthcare using appropriate technology and health promoting activities. Cultural sensitivity, **interprofessional collaboration** and community participation are further key features that enhance individual, family and community capacity to support parents and children in the **perinatal period** and early years. Primary healthcare recognises the influence of enabling and challenging social determinants of health in the lives of families, and seeks to identify modifications supporting health and wellness (McMurray & Clendon, 2015). Examples include having culturally sensitive healthcare services that are easily accessible in the community, either through home visiting or co-location on public transport routes, and having universally available free healthcare.

interprofessional collaboration Where two or more professional groups work together towards client-centred goals.

perinatal period The time of conception through to 12 months after a baby is born.

Case study 7.1: Nursing focus

Susan's story

Susan has recently been employed at a metropolitan Community Controlled Aboriginal Health Service as a maternal and child health nurse. She was previously working in an adult tertiary hospital. As a new staff member, Susan has been asked to participate in a reflective practice session with her manager to help her develop her practice role. During the conversation, she told her manager that she was becoming frustrated with mothers as they were not following her advice on how to address maternal and child health issues that she had identified, and were not compliant in attending clinic appointments

(Continued)

she made with herself and the service's medical practitioners. She told her manager that she wanted to make a difference to Aboriginal and Torres Strait Islander child and maternal health, but the clients were ignoring her strategies and treatment regimes.

CRITICAL REFLECTION QUESTIONS

- What are your responses to Susan's approach to clinical practice?
- What social determinants of health may be impacting on the clients?
- What key considerations does Susan need to take into account to effectively develop her practice role?
- How might Susan work in partnership with clients to create client-centred strategies?

Case study 7.2: Allied health focus

Abby's story

Abby is an experienced dietitian who has worked in a large regional hospital for the past 10 years. She has been chosen by her department to develop a regular outreach program to a rural community to provide nutrition advice, predominately to pregnant Aboriginal and Torres Strait Islander women. Despite her experience as an allied health professional, she has had limited opportunity to work with this group and is feeling quite anxious about this new role. Abby attended the hospital's compulsory cultural competency workshop 12 months ago and doesn't feel that this one-off workshop has adequately prepared her to successfully engage with her new clientele. The hospital has arranged for the new program to be run out of the local community health centre, but on her first couple of visits she has had a number of women not turn up. Speaking to other allied health professionals at her hospital, they also commented they get a lot of 'no shows' and just use the time to catch up on admin. Abby's line manager is keen for her to demonstrate the value of dietetics and wants to use Abby's new program as positive example where the hospital has improved healthcare for Aboriginal and Torres Strait Islander peoples. Abby is feeling pressure to deliver outcomes when she really feels she needs to spend time to better understand Aboriginal and Torres Strait Islander cultures and communities so that she can better support pregnant women to make positive nutritional choices.

Perinatal health and wellbeing

It is important to understand the relationship of pre-conceptual and perinatal health with positive birth outcomes and the developmental health of children and their families during the early years. Physical, cultural and psychosocial stressful experiences and environments at conception and during pregnancy can embed adverse biological changes in children's body systems, subsequently influencing people's abilities to maintain lifelong learning and health (Moore, Arefadib, Deery, Keyes & West, 2017). Recognising and reducing health disparities for Aboriginal and Torres Strait Islander parents and children is imperative for nursing and allied health practice. We will now consider more specific health and wellbeing through the antenatal, birthing and postnatal periods.

Case study 7.3: Nursing and allied health focus—an interprofessional approach

As registered nurses and allied health professionals, it is important to ensure clients feel that we are able to deliver culturally safe practices and work within culturally competent hospital and community health services. Consider the following case history for Mary, Tom and their family. Throughout the following sections, reflect on their worldviews and how culturally safe and culturally competent care may be perceived. What are the social determinants of health influencing their ability to maintain their health and wellbeing?

Mary and Tom's story

Mary and Tom are parents of an 18-month-old toddler, Emma, and three-year-old Jake. They live in an outer metropolitan suburb of an Australian capital

(Continued)

city and identify as an Australian Aboriginal family. Mary has attended an Aboriginal Community Controlled Health Service (ACCHS), which has a team of multi-disciplinary health professionals available for their clients. Mary has just had her third pregnancy confirmed at 10 weeks gestation.

Mary cares for her children full time and frequently looks after her sister's two children, aged six and eight, when she travels from a rural town for diabetes-related health appointments at the city's tertiary hospital. Mary states she is healthy apart from high blood glucose levels, which need further investigation. However, Mary is too tired and finds it difficult to attend the ACCHS as it is in the city and public transport is an issue in terms of frequency and managing her children. She can see a general practitioner in her area, but it is too far to walk, public transport remains an issue and she prefers the acceptance and welcome she receives at her local ACCHS. She walks to see her local child health nurse. She is a non-smoker and does not drink alcohol.

Tom's previous full-time employment at the local council has just been made into a casual position, which necessitates him using their only car three days a week to find additional work with a neighbouring council. Tom smokes 20 cigarettes a day and has approximately four standard drinks a week.

Emma and Jake are both reaching their developmental milestones, but Mary is concerned about their hearing. Jake has not been able to be properly assessed due to three episodes of otitis media in the past 12 months and Emma has a persistent runny nose. These have also affected their ability to have all their immunisations.

CRITICAL REFLECTION QUESTIONS

- What are the support opportunities that may facilitate Mary's wellness?
- What is the importance of family health in the antenatal period?

Antenatal period

Evidence suggests that Aboriginal and Torres Strait Islander women are at a greater risk of adverse pregnancy outcomes than other Australian women (Weetra et al., 2016; Gibson-Helm, Rumbold, Teede, Ranasinha, Bailie & Boyle, 2016; Kelly, West, Gamble, Sidebotham, Carson & Duffy, 2014). Common disparities include low birth weights, preterm birth, perinatal death and neural tube defects (Australian Institute of Health and Welfare, 2016; Leeds, Gourley, Laws, Zhang, Al-Yaman & Sullivan, 2007; Li, Zeki, Hilder & Sullivan, 2013; Bower, D'Antoine & Stanley, 2009). The higher presence of adverse outcomes is closely linked to increases in smoking and alcohol rates and poorer nutrition, alongside socio-economic disadvantage and barriers to accessing adequate antenatal care (Li et al., 2013; O'Leary, Halliday, Bartu, D'Antoine & Bower, 2013; McDermott, Campbell, Li & McCulloch, 2009).

It is evident that Aboriginal and Torres Strait Islander families experience higher rates of social health issues (Askew, Schluter, Spurling, Bond & Brown, 2013) and this can have a direct impact on maternal health and wellbeing (Weetra et al., 2016). Issues such as housing stress can affect women accessing antenatal care, which in turn limits opportunities to implement strategies to support healthy lifestyle choices that have positive outcomes for both mother and child (Weetra et al., 2016). There is also increasing evidence that family violence as well as other kinds of social adversities can have a significant influence on miscarriage, preterm birth and low birth weights (Shonkoff & Garner, 2012).

In 2011, 3.9% of women who gave birth in Australia identified as Aboriginal or Torres Strait Islander. Compared with other Australian women:

- They were on average five years younger than other mothers.
- They were 38.3% more likely to have a history of smoking and had lower rates of smoking cessation during pregnancy.
- They received fewer antenatal visits if they gave birth on or after 32 weeks.
- The average birth weight of their child was 187 grams lighter.
- Low-birth-weight rates were double that of other Australian women.
- Preterm births, which can be linked to adverse neonatal outcomes, were 5.7% more common.
- The maternal mortality ratio in 2008–12 was more than double (Li et al., 2013; Humphrey, Bonello, Chughtai, Macaldowie, Harris & Chambers, 2015).

It is evident that models of care to address these issues require a combination of high-quality clinical care alongside public health initiatives that address the modifiable social health risks (Weetra et al., 2016; Wong et al., 2011).

Balancing this is the many strengths Aboriginal and Torres Strait Islander peoples' cultures provide that support positive influences around pregnancy and childbirth, such as holistic approaches to wellbeing, supportive extended family networks and kinship, and a strong connection to country and culture (Clarke & Boyle, 2014). More work needs to be done to embed these strengths in maternal and child health programs at a community level.

High rates of alcohol consumption during pregnancy in some Aboriginal and Torres Strait Islander communities is leading to high a prevalence of conditions such as foetal alcohol syndrome (FAS) and partial foetal alcohol syndrome (pFAS; Mutch, Watkins & Bower, 2015). In a study undertaken by Fitzpatrick et al. (2014), they found that children born in the Fitzroy Valley, Western Australia, between 2002 and 2003 had the highest prevalence of FAS and pFAS worldwide. Teenage pregnancy also increases the chance of adverse outcomes (Chen et al., 2007). In a study undertaken by Steenkamp, Boyle, Kildea, Moore, Davies and Rumbold (2017) they found there were high rates of smoking and alcohol use in early pregnancy, particularly in urban indigenous teenagers.

With 19% of Aboriginal and Torres Strait Islander teens becoming pregnant before the age of 20, compared to 3% of non-Indigenous teens (Hilder, Zhichao, Parker, Jahan & Chambers, 2014), there needs to be a targeted focus on enhancing the wellbeing of teenagers through effective health promotion strategies (Steenkamp et al., 2017).

While there may be perceptions that these adverse outcomes primarily affect Aboriginal and Torres Strait Islander women in rural or remote areas, evidence suggests that urban Aboriginal and Torres Strait Islander populations also show marked disparities in pregnancy outcomes (Comino et al., 2012). It is therefore important that assumptions are not made that Aboriginal and Torres Strait Islander women living in urban areas have appropriate access and availability to the antenatal care they require.

CRITICAL REFLECTION QUESTIONS

- Why do you think these perceptions may exist?
- What are the challenges for women living in rural and remote areas?
- How do these compare with challenges for women such as Mary living in urban or outer urban areas?

Antenatal depression is also a significant issue for all pregnant women, with up to 20% of women internationally experiencing depression during pregnancy (Biaggi, Conroy, Pawlby & Pariante, 2015). While the risk factors associated with antenatal depression are multi-factorial, there are clear known contributors such as low socio-economic levels, low educational attainment, a history of depression and fewer antenatal visits (Leigh & Milgrom, 2008). Increased prevalence of these specific factors are evident within Aboriginal and Torres Strait Islander communities (Gausia et al., 2015). Routine screening both during pregnancy and postnatally using the Edinburgh Postnatal Depression Scale is recommended in Australia as standard practice (Australian Department of Health, 2009). However, studies have shown that Aboriginal and Torres Strait Islander women are not being routinely screened using the standard recommendations during pregnancy (Gausia et al., 2013; Gausia, Thompson, Nagel, Schierhout, Matthews & Bailie, 2015). In addition, standard screening tools may not adequately identify Aboriginal and Torres Strait Islander women 'at risk' of depression and anxiety during pregnancy due to differences in how mental disorders are perceived between Aboriginal and Torres Strait Islander communities and non-Indigenous communities (Gausia et al., 2015). Western views on mental health are grounded within an illness perspective, focusing on the individual and their interaction with the environment, whereas Aboriginal and Torres Strait Islander peoples have a more holistic standpoint incorporating social and emotional wellbeing and recognising the intersection of spirituality and connection to land, culture, family and community (Gausia et al., 2015). These different standpoints demonstrate how general standardised screening tools may not always be the most reliable approach to identify individuals 'at risk' of antenatal depression and anxiety within an Aboriginal and Torres Strait Islander population.

From a healthcare systems perspective, challenges exist in providing consistent, holistic and comprehensive antenatal care to Aboriginal and Torres Strait Islander women, not only in rural and remote areas but also within urban populations (Australian Health Ministers' Advisory Council, 2012). However, it is especially evident for Aboriginal and Torres Strait Islander women who live in remote locations, as they are often required to leave the family home and be transferred to larger regional settings to give birth (Corcoran, Catling & Homer, 2017; Gibson-Helm et al., 2016). Adequate antenatal care is critically important in addressing risks associated with adverse health outcomes for both the mother and the child (Gibson-Helm et al., 2016) and this can be achieved through fostering an environment that facilitates person-centred empowerment (Corcoran et al., 2017). Early identification and greater provision of pregnancy care, particularly around lifestyle-related factors, has shown to be effective in improving the health of Aboriginal and Torres Strait Islander mothers and therefore the health of children long term (Gibson-Helm et al., 2016). This can be further enhanced when models of care are based on a framework of continuous quality improvement and are incorporated into a culturally safe environment (Kildea, Stapleton, Murphy, Low & Gibbons, 2012; Wong et al., 2011; Gao et al., 2014).

It is well supported that Aboriginal and Torres Strait Islander women prefer to access maternity services that have Indigenous staff, as they have a shared understanding and cultural experience (Kelly et al., 2014). Effective antenatal care occurs when it is based on mutual trust, shared decision making and cultural sensitivity (Australian Health Ministers' Advisory Council, 2012). Being well supported and feeling safe during pregnancy and into the early months of a new born can directly impact on the social determinants of both mother and child (Buckskin et al., 2013). As such, maternity services that include Aboriginal and Torres Strait Islander staff have shown to have higher attendance rates, thus leading to better perinatal outcomes (Rumbold & Cunningham, 2008). In order to reduce disadvantage, there needs to be greater opportunities to enable Aboriginal and Torres Strait Islander peoples to enter the healthcare workforce, including an emphasis in midwifery and nursing to better support expectant mothers (Bryant, 2011). This can also be achieved through community-based and/or community-run programs or services that incorporate cultural knowledge and skills and are founded on partnership enabling more supportive and positive outcomes (Kildea, Gao, Rolfe, Josif, Bar-Zeev, Steenkamp & Barclay, 2016; Rumbold & Cunningham, 2008). In addition, tailoring services to meet the needs of Aboriginal and Torres Strait Islander women and providing flexible outreach services and transport options have been also shown to enhance positive experiences in antenatal care (Brown et al., 2015).

Figure 7.2 Improving antenatal outcomes for Aboriginal and Torres Strait Islander women

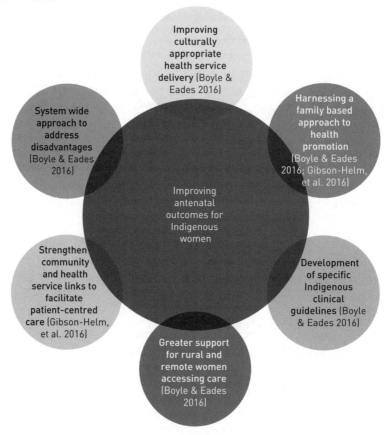

CRITICAL REFLECTION QUESTIONS

- As a health professional, how can you contribute to improving antenatal outcomes for Aboriginal and Torres Strait Islander women?
- What social determinants of health are impacting on Mary's ability to access antenatal care?
- Consider the culturally appropriate strategies you could use to engage Mary with health services to assist in her antenatal care.

Despite the challenges of providing appropriate antenatal care, there have been positive steps forward through the introduction of Aboriginal Community Controlled Health Services operating out of mainstream community health centres, delivering a range of maternal health services (Eades, 2004). These types of advancements have shown to decrease the prevalence of low birth weights and pre-term births

(Eades, 2004), while the 'Strong Women, Strong Babies, Strong Culture Program' values the cultural knowledge of senior women and their contribution to improving maternal and child health outcomes (Lowell, Kildea, Liddle, Cox & Paterson, 2015). However, models that incorporate Aboriginal Maternal Infant Care (AMIC) workers can also have challenges. These types of roles tend to be complex as they require staff to be skilled in both clinical and social models of health, with client relationships often extending into the community and beyond the visible role of the health system, which can be at odds with a Western health structure (Kirkham, Hoon, Rumbold & Moore, 2017). As such, AMIC workers can often find themselves isolated in a historical system that doesn't allow for flexibility in ways of working, potentially impacting on the sustainability of such programs (Kirkham et al., 2017).

While the development of maternal healthcare services specifically designed for Aboriginal and Torres Strait Islander women, including the role of AMIC workers, is a positive step forward in order to develop sustained outcomes, cultural competence must extend to all staff within the health organisation so that a greater appreciation of other ways of working across diverse populations (Kirkham et al., 2017) is realised.

CRITICAL REFLECTION QUESTIONS

- As a nursing or allied health professional engaged in maternal and child healthcare, what could you could do to develop a greater understanding of how AMIC workers approach supporting Aboriginal and Torres Strait Islander mothers?
- How could you liaise with an AMIC worker to support Mary and her family? Consider the options of home-visiting support and health-centre-based support.

Birthing

Healthy pregnancies and birth weights are enhanced when clients join in with pre-conceptual and antenatal care activities. These are crucial times for client engagement, with many vulnerable families not having the resources or understanding of the importance of linking with nurses and allied health staff. Research has identified that families are more likely to engage with these staff when the services are relationship based rather than content driven. Effective programs have a primary healthcare focus with client-centred goals and a partnership approach, where clients have choices of program strategies that are non-judgmental, demonstrate cultural sensitivity, provide help when they feel they need it, and are sustainable with long-term continuity of care (Centre for Community Child Health, 2010; Moore, McDonald, Sanjeevan & Price, 2012; Moore, 2015).

Being able to use traditional knowledge to guide birthing practices is pivotal to culturally safe practice. Birthing 'on country' is fundamentally important to Aboriginal culture and relationship to land. When Aboriginal mothers have no choice in having to give birth in hospitals away from home and their long-established supports, they can feel isolated, frightened and disempowered. These circumstances have the potential to lead to short- and long-term physical and psychosocial health outcomes (Kosiak, 2018).

Breastfeeding is vital for optimal growth, development and health (World Health Organization, 2011) and reduces the incidence of infectious diseases, allergies, asthma and otitis media (National Health and Medical Research Council, 2012). Traditional Aboriginal and Torres Strait Islander peoples' cultural practices encourage breastfeeding, but women may need additional support from nurses and allied health professionals to commence and maintain breastfeeding due to their anxiety, dislocation and feelings of not being supported. It is imperative to commence breastfeeding as soon as possible following birth to encourage and maintain breastfeeding, which also facilitates positive attachment and bonding between the mother and baby and helps reduce the risk of sudden infant death syndrome (McMurray & Clendon, 2015).

IMPLICATIONS FOR NURSING AND ALLIED HEALTH PRACTICE

Within your practice as registered nurses and allied health professionals, what do you see as the factors impacting on perinatal mental health for Mary? Consider both enabling and risk factors. How could a primary healthcare approach to practice enhance Mary's pregnancy and the health and wellbeing of the whole family?

Postnatal care

Similarly to Aboriginal and Torres Strait Islander mothers, the overall health of Aboriginal and Torres Strait Islander children has been shown to be poorer compared to non-Indigenous Australians (Brewster & Morris, 2015). The first couple of months of life is often the most vulnerable for a baby and is the most critical time for access to appropriate primary healthcare services (Hill, Kirkwood & Edmond, 2004). However, evidence suggests that not all Aboriginal and Torres Strait Islander babies are receiving the recommended scheduled primary healthcare, despite the availability of high-quality maternity services (Eades & Stanley, 2013). In addition to low birth weights and foetal alcohol syndrome that has been noted (Australian Institute of Health and Welfare 2016; Mutch et al., 2015), a number of other health conditions have high prevalence rates in Aboriginal and Torres Strait Islander children (Brewster & Morris, 2015), discussed below.

Sudden infant death syndrome (SIDS)

It has been shown that Aboriginal and Torres Strait Islander infants have a higher rate of SIDS than non-Indigenous infants (Sayers & Boyle, 2010). Risk factors include sleeping prone, higher rates of smoking during pregnancy and sharing a bed (Brewster & Morris, 2015).

Diarrhoeal disease

There is a strong link between diarrhoeal disease and malnutrition within Aboriginal and Torres Strait Islander child populations (Brewster & Morris, 2015). The causes of this are complex and multi-factorial, but can be linked to bacterial contamination and increased incidence of infestations and intestinal infections, as well as environmental contamination (Brewster, 2002).

Meningitis

Studies have shown that there was a fivefold increase of Aboriginal and Torres Strait Islander children contracting H. influenza type b (Hib) meningitis and a sixfold increase in pneumococcal meningitis compared to non-Indigenous children (Bower, Payne, Condon, Hendrie, Harris & Henderson, 1994; King & Richmond, 2004). In these studies they also found that there were significantly higher rates of severe neurological damage (Bower et al., 1994; King & Richmond, 2004) as a result of contracting meningitis.

Rheumatic fever

Significant morbidity due to rheumatic fever and rheumatic heart disease is still evident in Aboriginal and Torres Strait Islander populations, especially in northern Australia (Currie & Brewster, 2002). This may be related to ongoing poor living conditions and overcrowding, with exposure to group A streptococci (Webb & Wilson, 2013). Children who present with acute rheumatic fever are also at risk of developing permanent disability due to carditis and arthritis and should be managed through antibiotic therapy as soon as possible (Brewster & Morris, 2015).

Respiratory diseases, including otitis media

It is common for Aboriginal and Torres Strait Islander children to have severe and frequent bacterial and viral infections (Bailey, Maclennan, Morris, Kruske, Brown & Chang, 2009). Otitis media is a common condition seen in Aboriginal and Torres

Strait Islander children, and is typically seen at an earlier age and lasts longer than in non-Indigenous paediatric populations (Jervis-Bardy, Sanchez & Carney, 2014). In the most severe cases the infection begins in the first few weeks of life and often results in perforation of the tympanic membrane, resulting in hearing loss (Leach & Morris, 2001) leading to ongoing issues with speech and language as well as success in education.

Malnutrition

Evidence suggests that poor nutrition postnatally has been directly related to irreversible damage to areas such as neurological, immune and physical development (Grantham-McGregor, Walker & Chang, 2000). However, poor nutrition is often interrelated with other facets of disadvantage such as economic, psychological and social inequalities (Ritte, Panozzo, Johnston, Agerholm, Kvernmo, Rowely & Arabena, 2016). It is therefore critically important to ensure that there is a focus on the first 1000 days in Aboriginal and Torres Strait Islander children due to the increased rates of vulnerability seen (Ou, Chan, Garrett & Hillman, 2010). However, solely relying on nutritional interventions is unlikely to result in significant change; rather, the focus needs to consider the larger context of disadvantage for these children (Ritte et al., 2016).

Scabies, impetigo and trachoma

Scabies, impetigo and trachoma are common infectious conditions that are underpinned by challenging environmental conditions and social determinants of health, such as overcrowding in homes and lack of adequate sanitation. Scabies is a parasitic infection of the skin that is very prevalent in Aboriginal and Torres Strait Islander communities in northern Australia. Scabies mites are located under the skin surface, predominately in hands, feet, genitalia and scalp, with the resulting wounds becoming itchy and causing secondary bacterial infections. Long-term health trajectories for this condition include pain, scarring, and recurring infections, which predispose to rheumatic fever, and rheumatic heart and renal diseases (Department of Health, 2018; Hardy, Engelman & Steer, 2017).

Impetigo is a milder bacterial skin infection caused by staphylococcus or streptococcus bacteria and is also common in school communities in northern Australia. Impetigo manifests as itchy sores on the skin, typically commencing as blisters before they burst and suppurate (Royal Children's Hospital, n.d; Bowen, Tong, Chatfield & Carapetis, 2014).

Trachoma is usually found in communities experiencing hot, dry conditions and is caused by the *Chlamydia trachomatis* bacterial infection. The most common age for the infection is in children aged two to three years, but may be identified in older children up to early adolescence (Australian Indigenous HealthInfoNet, 2013). The inside of the eyelid can become scarred, causing the eyelashes to turns inward and rub against the cornea. The consequences of this irritation are pain, corneal scarring and visual difficulties with ultimate blindness (World Health Organization, 2019). Sustainable management of scabies, impetigo and trachoma require not only screening and medication but also fundamental recognition of the impact of adverse social determinants of health on long-term clinical and social outcomes (Lowitja Institute, n.d.; Currie & Carapetis, 2001).

Early opportunities to connect with health services have positive benefits for both mother and child. Developing models of care for children that focus on a more holistic approach and address social disadvantage through incorporating an emphasis on protecting culture and identity are likely to realise positive health and wellbeing outcomes in future generations (Hartley, 1995). As such, strategies that are community controlled and facilitate change by empowering families are likely to have the greatest chance of making a difference (Commonwealth of Australia, 2013). Approaches that empower parents through partnership and peer support have also shown to be successful (Munns & Walker, 2015). Models of care such as targeted support and care coordination from hospital also have the potential to enhance the provision of primary care for infants while supporting the whole family during this vulnerable period (McAullay et al., 2016; Goyal, Teeters & Ammerman, 2013).

In a model proposed by Ritte et al. (2016), key elements were identified to facilitate positive outcomes for children within the first 1000 days. These are outlined in Table 7.1.

Table 7.1 Key elements to facilitate positive outcomes for children within the first 1000 days

Key elements	Examples
Community governance	Engage Aboriginal and Torres Strait Islander peoples to be involved in co-design, co-implementation and co-knowledge translation of program outcomes and research through all levels of government.
Family environment	Focus on a strengths-based approach that enhances family relationships within the broader context and cultural links. Facilitate a shift towards maximising protective factors in families rather than a reliance on child maternal health services.
Increasing antenatal and early years' engagement	Focus on a whole-of-service approach in program design. Develop strategies to increase participation of men during the transition to fatherhood. Investigate innovative approaches that focus on wellbeing outside of the health context to improve family circumstances.
Service use and provision	Ensure that there is capacity building with parents, the extended family and the workforce to support the diversity among nations. Broaden the focus of programs from clinical service delivery to improving access to services through a client-centred approach within programs focused on the first 1000 days.

Source: Ritte et al. (2016).

Role of the community child health nurse

In order to reduce risks of poor health conditions, it is important for families to engage with community child health nurses early in the postnatal period. These nurses have a broad role, including home visiting, early identification of and intervention for physical and psychosocial issues, one-to-one and group client contact, and interprofessional allied health case management (Borrow, Munns & Henderson, 2011). Of emerging interest is the partnership approach between child health nurses, peer support workers and families to facilitate culturally safe support for Aboriginal and Torres Strait Islander parents through community-based activities and/or home visiting. Peer support workers are local community members with established neighbourhood networks and a willingness to offer non-professional psychosocial support to families with young children (Munns, Toye, Hegney, Kickett, Marriott & Walker, 2018). This contrasts with the professional practice of Aboriginal health workers who work to provide direct or collaborative care with nurses and allied health professionals (Drummond, 2018).

Developmental health

Evidence suggests that by the time Aboriginal and Torres Strait Islander children enter school, almost half have signs of developmental vulnerability (Brinkman et al., 2012). This often results in poor literacy and numeracy outcomes that continue throughout a child's school years (DeBortoli & Thompson, 2010) and result in increased rates of leaving school early and not completing Year 12 (Australian Institute of Health and Welfare, 2011). Furthermore, this path often directly links to further disadvantage as an adult due to limited education, unemployment and reduced life opportunities impacting on overall health and wellbeing (Australian Bureau of Statistics, 2010).

Studies have also shown that poor perinatal and socio-demographic factors can also impact a child's educational performance at school (Malacova, Li, Blair, Leonard, de Klerk & Stanley, 2008) as there is a strong link between delayed early childhood development and social disadvantage (Hanley et al., 2018; Nicholson, Lucas, Berthelsen & Wake, 2012) (see Figure 7.3). Nutrition plays a significant role, especially within the first two years of life, to allow children to reach their full potential (Wise, 2013). In a study undertaken by Guthridge, Lin, Silburn, Shu, Qin, McKenzie and Lynch (2015), they found that when comparing Aboriginal and Torres Strait Islander children and non-Indigenous children in the Northern Territory, Aboriginal and Torres Strait Islander children who had low birth weights and evidence of maternal smoking had poorer educational outcomes and were at higher risk of developmental, cognitive and health problems compared to non-Indigenous children (Guthridge et al., 2015).

Figure 7.3 Trajectories for adverse prenatal outcomes

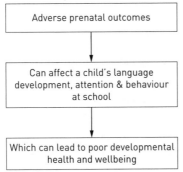

Source: Haung and Haung (2012).

CRITICAL REFLECTION QUESTIONS

- Reflect on the health and wellbeing of Mary and Tom's family. What do you see as their physical and psychosocial strengths during the birthing and postnatal periods? What are their vulnerabilities?
- How could nurses and allied health professionals work in partnership with Mary and Tom to develop appropriate support and strategies to address these vulnerabilities. How could the family's strengths be utilised?

The family environment also has a strong impact on early childhood development, with the physical or mental conditions of parents having a lasting influence on their relationships with their children (Wise, 2013). In addition, the over-representation of Aboriginal and Torres Strait Islander children under the scrutiny of government departments concerned with child services increases their vulnerability and has a negative effect on wellbeing during this age period (Wise, 2013).

Early childhood vulnerability is not confined to rural or remote populations, with urban Aboriginal and Torres Strait Islander children also showing similar, and in some cases higher, rates of poor health outcomes (Eades, Bailey, Williamson, Craig & Redman, 2010). In a study undertaken by Gardner et al. (2016), they found that urban Aboriginal and Torres Strait Islander children had increased health needs, complex family situations and increased levels of developmental risk. Therefore, it is important that we do not make assumptions that the overall health status is better for urban children just because they live in the cities.

Early detection and intervention is critically important in reducing the long-term impacts of developmental problems in children (Simpson, D'Aprano, Tayler, Toon Khoo & Highfold, 2016). This is especially important for those children already showing some signs of developmental delay (Guralnick, 2011). In contrast, the longer developmental issues are left without intervention, the greater the risk of long-standing implications for the child as they grow older (Guevara et al., 2013).

Evidence suggests that enhancing children's health, wellbeing and development in the early years, alongside high-quality education, has long-term positive effects (Gluckman, Hanson, Cooper & Thornburg, 2008; Graham & Power, 2004). In addition, healthy nutrition, adequate psychosocial stimulation and responsive parenting have been shown to have protective benefits that can limit the impact of early disadvantage (Landry, Smith, Swank, Assel & Vellet, 2001).

It is well appreciated that the social conditions of young children can have a direct impact on overall health and development (Pillas, Marmot, Naicker, Goldblatt, Morrison, & Pilkhart, 2014). Alongside this, early childhood also provides the greatest opportunities for early interventions to be instigated to improve developmental outcomes and reverse potential trends (Moss, Harper & Silburn, 2015). In response, there has been a focus by the Australian Government on increasing funding towards early childhood development to decrease the social and economic disadvantage seen in Aboriginal and Torres Strait Islander populations (Council of Australian Governments, 2008). In a study undertaken by Guthridge, Lin, Silburn, Shu Qin, McKenzie and Lynch (2016), they found that children not attending childcare or preschool programs had an increased risk of vulnerability. This finding supports approaches to increase the accessibility and availability of Aboriginal and Torres Strait Islander children attending preschool, especially in remote areas (Council of Australian Governments, 2008). As a result, a number of new models have been instigated to assist in enhancing the developmental outcomes of young Aboriginal and Torres Strait Islander children.

Innovative approaches such as early childhood programs that embed cultural context at a local level through a shared understanding of priorities, needs and strengths have been shown to make meaningful contributions to enhancing Aboriginal and Torres Strait Islander children's potential during early childhood (Wise, 2013). Preschool programs that provide appropriate support mechanisms that focus on language and education matched to the individual child's needs have also shown positive outcomes (Guthridge et al., 2016). Other targeted programs, such as the Preschool Readiness Program (PRP), which are founded in a collaborative framework and focus on preschool attendance alongside health and developmental checks, not only support the child's educational needs but also foster better communication with families while enabling early referral pathways to other service providers (Moss, Harper & Silburn, 2015). The Brighter Futures Program is another example of a specific early-intervention program that aims to prevent vulnerable children from entering child protection by providing access to interventions and support to families at risk (Department of Community Services, 2012).

Despite the positive benefits of such approaches, these types of programs still have a number of challenges as they often rely on commitment and collaboration from outside health and education organisations, which are still tending to work in a fragmented and unilateral service delivery model (Moss, Harper & Silburn, 2015). In order to ensure the long-term sustainability of such programs, commitment to ongoing dialogue between organisations is needed, as well as increased understanding of the continuing barriers for Aboriginal and Torres Strait Islander children to participate in such programs (Moss, Harper & Silburn, 2015).

IMPLICATIONS FOR NURSING AND ALLIED HEALTH PRACTICE

Within your roles as registered nurses and allied health professionals, what are the enabling and challenging factors influencing the developmental health and wellbeing of the children in Tom and Mary's biological and extended family? How could you work interprofessionally and in partnership with this family to develop strategies to address the challenges?

CRITICAL REFLECTION QUESTIONS

- What are the key nursing and allied health practice considerations for Tom and Mary's family?
- What elements within nursing and allied health practice could be addressed to develop effective cultural safety and cultural competence for this family and their community?

Conclusion

Culturally responsive healthcare in the early years is imperative to enable meaningful and individual health outcomes within Aboriginal and Torres Strait Islander communities. This chapter has introduced key concepts, perspectives and models of practice that will support child and maternal development in the early years.

SUMMARY

Throughout this chapter, you have been encouraged to consider concepts of Aboriginal and Torres Strait Islander peoples' maternal and child health and wellbeing. You have been able to reflect on the worldviews of Aboriginal and Torres Strait Islander parents and what is important for them to enable engagement with nursing and allied health professionals.

Learning concept 1

Explore concepts of Aboriginal and Torres Strait Islander peoples' maternal and child health and wellbeing: It is important to understand how Aboriginal and Torres Strait Islander peoples' holistic view of health impacts on their parenting practices, thereby influencing children's growth and development. Physical, cultural, spiritual and social elements are central to maternal health and wellbeing.

Learning concept 2

Identify the importance of Indigenous Australian cultural competence for maternal and child health: Nursing and allied health strategies need to be perceived as culturally safe for parents in the perinatal period and with children in the early years. Culturally competent health professionals will enable the delivery of culturally safe care.

Learning concept 3

Identify and explore social determinants of health impacting on Aboriginal and Torres Strait Islander peoples' perinatal health and the early years: Understanding the social determinants of health is important for health professionals in the delivery of care. The social determinants of health can have a lasting impact on individuals and families. Sustainable programs that facilitate wellness can result in improved health outcomes.

Learning concept 4

Identify and explore interprofessional skills for working in culturally competent partnership with Aboriginal and Torres Strait Islander individuals, families and communities in the perinatal period and early years: Interprofessional skills that are constructed within a strengths-based culturally competent framework enable health professionals to facilitate meaningful relationships with consumers of healthcare that facilitate the health and wellness of the family.

Learning concept 5

Identify and explore the roles of nurses and allied health professionals working with Aboriginal and Torres Strait Islander families with young children: Registered nurses and allied health professionals need to ensure clients feel that they are able to deliver culturally safe practices within culturally competent hospital and community health services. This includes identifying client strengths, and using a primary healthcare approach and interprofessional practice, all of which underpin culturally competent practice.

REVISION QUESTIONS

1. Why do nursing and allied health practitioners need to consider the impact of social determinants of health on maternal and child health?
2. How can primary healthcare principles and strategies strengthen nursing and allied healthcare practice, particularly for Aboriginal and Torres Strait Islander maternal and child health?
3. Taking into account their social determinants of health, how can parents and extended family members maintain their children's developmental health and wellbeing? What culturally safe and culturally competent strategies could be facilitated by nursing and allied health professionals?
4. How could you work interprofessionally and in partnership with clients to facilitate a healthy pregnancy and culturally safe birth?
5. How can interprofessional practice for nursing and allied health professionals enhance the mental health of clients during the perinatal period?

FURTHER READINGS/ADDITIONAL RESOURCES

Beyond Blue. (2011). Aboriginal and Torres Strait Islander perinatal mental health. A guide for primary care health professionals. Retrieved http://resources.beyondblue.org.au/prism/file?token=BL/1081

REFERENCES

Askew, D. A., Schluter, P. J., Spurling, G. K. P., Bond, C. J. R., & Brown, A. D. H. (2013). Urban Aboriginal and Torres Strait Islander children's exposure to stressful events: A cross sectional study. *Medical Journal of Australia*, 199(1), 42-45.

Australian Bureau of Statistics. (2010). *The health welfare of Australia's Aboriginal and Torres Strait Islander peoples*. ABS Catalogue no. 4704.0. Canberra: ABS.

Australian Department of Health. (2009). Framework for the National Perinatal Depression Initiative 2008–09 to 2012–13. *Health TAGoDo*. Retrieved from http://www.health.gov.au/internet/publications/publishing.nsf/Content/mental-pubs-fperinat-toc~mental-pubs-f-perinat-fra

Australian Health Ministers' Advisory Council. (2012). *Clinical practice guidelines: Antenatal care—module 1*. Canberra: Australian Government Department of Health and Ageing.

Australian Indigenous HealthInfoNet. (2013). *Trachoma*. Retrieved from https://healthinfonet.ecu.edu.au/learn/health-topics/eye-health/trachoma

Australian Institute of Health and Welfare. (2016). *Australia's mothers and babies 2014 in brief*. Perinatal statistics series No. 32. Cat no. PER 87. Canberra: Author.

Australian Institute of Health and Welfare. (2011). *The health and welfare of Australia's Aboriginal and Torres Strait Islander people: An overview*. Cat. No. IHW 42. Canberra: AIHW.

Australian Institute of Health and Welfare & Australian Institute of Family Studies. (2013). *Strategies and practices for promoting the social and emotional wellbeing of Aboriginal and Torres Strait Islander people*. Canberra: Australian government. Retrieved from https://www.aihw. gov.au/getmedia/1c9d820f-4bf4-437d-8b15-dec682b9774c/ctgc-rs19.pdf.aspx?inline=true

Bailey, E. J., Maclennan, C., Morris, P. S., Kruske, S. G., Brown, N., & Chang, A. B. (2009). Risks of severity and readmission of Indigenous and non-Indigenous children hospitalised for bronchiolitis. *Journal of Paediatric Child Health*, *45*, 593-597.

Biaggi, A., Conroy, S., Pawlby, S., & Pariante, C. M. (2016). Identifying the women at risk of antenatal anxiety and depression: A systematic review. *J Affect Disord*, *191*, 62-77. doi: 10.1016/j.jad.2015.11.014

Borrow, S., Munns, A., & Henderson, S. (2011). Community-based child health nurses: An exploration of current practice. *Contemporary Nurse*, *40*(1), 71-86.

Bowen, A. C., Tong, S. Y. T., Chatfield, M. D., & Carapetis, J. R. (2014). The microbiology of impetigo in Indigenous children: Associations between Streptococcus pyogenes, Staphylococcus aureus, scabies, and nasal carriage. *BMC Infectious Diseases*, *14*, 727. doi:10.1186/s12879-014-0727-5

Bower, C., D'Antoine, H., & Stanley, F. J. (2009). Neural tube defects in Australia: Trends in encephaloceles and other neural tube defects before and after promotion of folic acid supplementation and voluntary food fortification. *Birth Defects Res Part A Clin Mol Teratol*, *85*(4), 269-273.

Bower, C., Payne, J., Condon, R., Hendrie, D., Harris, A., & Henderson, R. (1994). Sequelae of Haemophilus influeznae type b meningitis in Aboriginal and non-Aboriginal children under 5 years. *Journal of Paediatric Child Health*, *30*, 393-397.

Boyle, J., & Eades, S. (2016). Closing the gap in Aboriginal women's reproductive health: Some progress, but still a long way to go. *Aust N Z J Obstet Gynaecol*, *56*(3), 223-224.

Brewster, D. R., & Morris, P. S. (2015). Indigenous child health: Are we making progress? *Journal of Paediatrics and Child Health*, *51*, 40-47.

Brewster, D. R. (2002). Dehydration in acute gastroenteritis. *Journal of Paediatric Child Health*, 38, 219-222.

Brinkman, S. A., Gialamas, A., & Rahman, A. Mittinty, M. N., Gregory, T. A., Silburn, S., … Lynch, J. W. (2012). Jurisdictional, socio-economic and gender equalities in child health and development: Analysis of a national census of 5-year olds in Australia. *BMJ Open*, e001075.

Brown, S. J., Weetra, D., Glover, K., Buckskin, M., Ah Kit, J., Leane, C., … Yelland, J. (2015). Improving Aboriginal women's experiences of maternity care: Results of the Aboriginal Families Study. *Birth*, *42*(1), 27-37.

Bryant, R. (2011). How can the nursing and midwifery help close the gap in Indigenous indicators? *Contemporary Nurse*, *37*(1), 8-9.

Buckskin, M., Ah Kit, J., Glover, K., Mitchell, A., Miller, R., Weetra, D., … Brown, S. J. (2013). Aboriginal Families Study: Social history of an Australian population-based study that aimed to keep community and policy goals in mind right from the start. *Int. J. Equity Health Care*, *12*, 41.

Centre for Community Child Health. (2010). *Engaging marginalised and vulnerable families*. CCCH Policy Brief No. 18. Parkville: Centre for Community Child Health, Royal Children's Hospital. Retrieved from http://www.rch.org.au/emplibrary/ccch/PB18_Vulnerable_families.pdf

Chen, X. K., Wen, S.W., Fleming, N., Demissie, K., Rhodes, G.G., & Walker, M. (2007). Teenage pregnancy and adverse birth outcomes: A large population retrospective cohort study. *International Journal of Epidemiology*, *32*(2), 368-373.

https://doi.org/10.1093/ije/dyl284

Clarke, M., & Boyle, J. (2014). Antenatal care for Aboriginal and Torres Strait Islander women. *Aust Fam Physician*, *43*(1), 20-24.

Comino, E., Knight, J., Webster, V., Jackson Pulver, L., Jalaludin, B., Harris, E., ... Harris, M. (2012). Risk and protective factors for pregnancy outcomes for urban Aboriginal and non-Aboriginal mothers and infants: The Gudaga cohort. *Maternal and Child Health Journal*, *16*(3), 569-578. doi:10.1007/s10995-011-0789-6

Commonwealth of Australia. (2013). *National Aboriginal and Torres Strait Islander health plan 2013–2023*. Canberra: Australian Government.

Corcoran, P., Catling, C., & Homer, C. (2017). Models of midwifery care for Indigenous women and babies: A meta-synthesis. *Women and Birth*, *30*, 77-86.

Council of Australian Governments. (2008). *National partnership agreement for indigenous early childhood development*. Canberra: COAG.

Currie, B. J., & Brewster, D. R. (2002). Rheumatic fever in Aboriginal children. *Journal of Paediatric Child Health*, *38*, 223-225.

Currie, B. J., & Carapetis, J. R. (2001). Skin infections and infestations in Aboriginal communities in northern Australia. *Australian Journal of Dermatology*, *41*(3), 139-143. https://doi.org/10.1046/j.1440-0960.2000.00417.x

DeBortoli, L., & Thomson, S. (2010). *Contextual factors that influence the achievement of Australia's Indigenous students: Results from PISA 2000–2006* (p. 7). OECD Programme for International Student Assessment (PISA).

Department of Community Services. (2012). *Brighter futures service provision guidelines*. Sydney: Department of Community Services.

Department of Health. (2018). *Indigenous health—crusted scabies.* Retrieved from http://www.health.gov.au/internet/budget/publishing.nsf/Content/budget2018-factsheet16.htm

Drummond, A. (2018). Working with Aboriginal and Torres Strait Islander health workers and health practitioners. In O. Best & B. Fredericks (Eds.), *Yatdjuligin: Aboriginal and Torres Strait Islander nursing and midwifery care* (2nd ed., pp. 155-178). Cambridge: Cambridge University Press.

Eades, S. J., & Stanley, F. J. (2013). Improving the health of First Nation children in Australia. *Medical Journal of Australia*, *199*, 12-13.

Eades, S. T., Bailey, S., Williamson, A. B., Craig, J. C., & Redman, S. (2010). The health of urban Aboriginal people: Insufficient data to close the gap. *Medical Journal of Australia*, *193*, 521-524.

Eades, S. (2004). Maternal and child health care services: Actions in the primary health care setting to improve the health of Aboriginal and Torres Strait Islander women of childbearing age, infants and young children. Canberra: Commonwealth of Australia.

Fenton, A., Walsh, K., Wong, S., & Cumming, T. (2015). Using strengths-based approaches in the early years practice and research. *International Journal of Early Childhood*, 47(1), 27-52.

Fitzpatrick, J. P., Latimer, J., Carter, M., Oscar, J., Ferreira, M. L., Carmichael Olson, H., … Elliot, E. J. (2015) Prevalence of fetal alcohol syndrome in a population-based sample of children living in remote Australia: The Lililwan Project. *Journal of Paediatrics and Child Health*, 51, 450-457. doi:10.1111/jpc.12814

Gao, Y., Gold, L., Josif, C., Bar-Zeev, S., Steenkamp, M., Barclay, L., … Kildea, S. (2014). A cost-consequences analysis of a midwifery group practice for Aboriginal mothers and infants in the top end of the Northern Territory, Australia. *Midwifery*, 30(4), 447-455.

Gardner, S., Woolfenden, S., Callaghan, L., Allende, T., Winters, J., Wong, G., … Zwi, K. (2016). Picture of the health status of Aboriginal children living in an urban setting of Sydney. *Australian Health Review*, 40, 337-344. http://dx.doi.org/10.1071/AH14259

Gausia, K., Thompson, S., Nagel, T., Rumbold, A., Connors, C., Matthews, V., … Bailie, R. (2013). Antenatal emotional wellbeing screening in Aboriginal and Torres Strait Islander primary health care services in Australia. *Contemp Nurse*, 46, 73-82.

Gausia, K., Thompson, S. C., Nagel, T., Schierhout, G., Matthews, V., & Bailie, R. (2015). Risk of antenatal psychosocial distress in indigenous women and its management at primary health care centres in Australia. *General Hospital Psychiatry*, 37(4), 335-339.

Gibson-Helm, M., Rumbold, A. R., Teede, H. J., Ranasinha, S., Bailie, R. S., & Boyle, J. A. (2016). Improving the provision of pregnancy care for Aboriginal and Torres Strait islander women: A continuous quality improvement initiative. *BMC Pregnancy and Childbirth*, 16. doi:http://dx.doi.org/10.1186/s12884-016-0892-1

Gluckman, P., Hanson, M. A., Cooper, C., & Thornburg, K. L. (2008). Effect of in utero and early-life conditions on adult health and disease. *New England Journal of Medicine*, 359, 61-73. doi:10.1056/NEJMra0708473

Goyal, N. K., Teeters, A., & Ammerman, R. T. (2013). Home visiting and outcomes of preterm infants: A systematic review. *Pediatrics*, 132, 13-17.

Graham, H., & Power, C. (2004). Childhood disadvantage and health inequalities: A framework for policy based on lifecourse research. *Child Care Health Development*, 30, 671-8.

Grantham-McGregor, S. M., Walker, S. P., & Chang, S. (2000). Nutritional deficiencies and later behavioural development. *Proceedings of the Nutritional Society*, 59, 47-54.

Guevara, J. P., Gerdes, M., Localio, R., Huang, Y. V., Pinto-Martin, J., Minkovitz, C. S., … Pati, S. (2012). Effectiveness of developmental screening in an urban setting. *Pediatrics*, 131(1), 30-37.

Guralnick, M. J. (2011). Why early intervention works: A systems perspective. *Infants and Young Children*, 24(1), 6.

Guthridge, S., Lin, L., Silburn, S., Shu Qin, L., McKenzie, J., & Lynch. J. (2015). Impact of perinatal health and socio-demographic factors on school education outcomes: A population study of Indigenous and non-indigenous children in the Northern Territory. *Journal of Paediatrics and Child Health*. 51, 778-786.

Guthridge, S., Lin, L., Silburn, S., Shu Qin, L., McKenzie, J., & Lynch. J. (2016). Early influences on developmental outcomes among children, at age 5, in Australia's Northern Territory. *Early Childhood Research Quarterly*, 35, 124-134.

Hampton, R., & Toombs, M. (Eds.). *Indigenous Australians and health. The wombat in the room.* South Melbourne: Oxford University Press.

Hanley, M., Falster, K., Chambers, G., Lynch, J., Banks, E., Homaira, N., ... Jorm, L. (2018). Gestational age and child development at age five in population-based cohort of Australian Aboriginal and non-Aboriginal children. *Paediatric and Perinatal Epidemiology, 32*, 114-125.

Hardy, M., Engelman, D., & Steer, A. (2017). Scabies: A clinical update. *Australian Family Physician, 46*(5), 264-268.

Hartley, R. (1995). *Families and cultural diversity in Australia* (pp. 48-69). Canberra: Australian Institute of Family Studies.

Hilder, L., Zhichao, Z., Parker, M., Jahan, S., & Chambers, G. (2014). *Australia's mothers and babies 2012.* Canberra: National Perinatal Epidemiology and Statistics Unit.

Hill, Z., Kirkwood, B., & Edmond, K. (2004). *Family and community practices that promote child survival, growth and development: A review of the evidence.* Geneva: World Health Organization.

Humphrey, M., Bonello, M., Chughtai, A., Macaldowie, A., Harris, K., & Chambers, G. (Eds.). (2015). *Maternal deaths in Australia 2008–2012.* Canberra: Australian Institute of Health and Welfare.

Huang, J. H., & Huang, H., J. (2012). Inattention and development of toddlers born preterm and with low birth weights. *Kaolhsiung Journal of Medical Science, 28*, 390-396. doi:10.1016/j-kms.2012.02.006

Jervis-Bardy, J., Sanchez, L., & Carney, A. S. (2014). Otitis media in Indigenous Australian children: A review of epidemiology and risk factors. *Journal of Laryngology & Otology, 128*(Suppl. SI), S16-S27.

Kelly, J., West, R., Gamble, J., Sidebotham, M., Carson, V., & Duffy, E. (2014). 'She knows how we feel': Australian Aboriginal and Torres Strait Islander childbearing women's experience of continuity of care with an Australian Aboriginal and Torres Strait Islander midwifery student. *Women Birth, 27*, 157-162.

Kildea, S., Gao, Y., Rolfe, M., Josif, C., Bar-Zeev, S., Steenkamp, M., & Barclay, L. (2016). Remote links: redesigning maternity care for Aboriginal women from remote communities in Northern Australia—a comparative cohort study. *Midwifery.* 34, 47-57.

Kildea, S., Stapleton, H., Murphy, R., Low, N. B., & Gibbons, K. (2012). The Murri clinic: A comparative retrospective study of an antenatal clinic developed for Aboriginal and Torres Strait Islander women. *BMC Pregnancy and Childbirth, 12*, 159.

King, B. A., & Richmond, P. (2004). Pneumococcal meningitis in Western Australian children: Epidemiology, microbiology, and outcome. *Journal of Paediatric Child Health, 40*, 611-615.

Kirkham, R., Hoon, E., Rumbold., & Moore, V. (2017). Understanding the role of Australian Aboriginal maternal infant care workers: Bringing a cultural dimension to a critique of the ideal worker concept. *Community, Work & Family, 21*(4), 393-409. doi:10.1080/13668803.20 17.1304893

Kosiak, M. (2018). Midwifery practices and Aboriginal and Torres Strait Islander women: Urban and regional perspectives. In O. Best & B. Fredericks (Eds.), *Yatdjuligin: Aboriginal and Torres Strait Islander nursing and midwifery care* (2nd ed., pp. 113-137). Cambridge: Cambridge University Press.

Landry, S., Smith, K. E., Swank, P. R., Assel, M. A., & Vellet, S. (2001). Does early responsive parenting have a special importance for children's development or is consistency across childhood necessary? *Developmental Psychology*. 37: 387-403.

Leach, A. J., & Morris, P. S. (2001). Perspectives on infective ear disease in indigenous Australian children. *Journal of Paediatric Child Health*, *37*, 529-530.

Leeds, K., Gourley, M., Laws, P., Zhang, J., Al-Yaman, F., & Sullivan, E. (2007). *Indigenous mothers and their babies, Australia 2001–2004* (Perinatal statistics series, vol. 19). Canberra: Australian Institute of Health and Welfare.

Leigh, B., & Milgrom, J. (2008). Risk factors for antenatal depression, postnatal depression and parenting stress. *BMC Psychiatry*, *8*, 24.

Li, Z., Zeki, R., Hilder, L., & Sullivan, E. A. (2013). *Australia's mothers and babies 2011* (Perinatal statistics series, vol. 28). Canberra: Australian Institute of Health and Welfare.

Lowell, A., Kildea, S., Liddle, M., Cox, B., & Paterson, B. (2015). Supporting Aboriginal knowledge and practice in health care: Lessons from qualitative evaluation of Strong Women, Strong Babies, Strong Culture program. *BMC*, *15*, 19. doi:10.1186/s12884-015-0433-3

Lowitja Institute. (n.d.). *Skin infections and infestations in Aboriginal communities in northern Australia*. Retrieved from https://www.lowitja.org.au/skin-infections-and-infestations-aboriginal-communities-northern-australia

Malacova, E., Li, J., Blair, E., Leonard, H., de Klerk, N., & Stanley, F. (2008). Association of birth outcomes and maternal, school and neighbourhood characteristics with subsequent numeracy achievement. *American Journal of Epidemiology*, *168*, 21-29.

McAullay, D., McAuley, K., Marriot, R., Pearson, G., Jacoby, P., Ferguson, C., ... Edmond, K. (2016). Improving access to primary care for Aboriginal babies in Western Australia: A study protocol for a randomised controlled trial. *Trials*, *17*, 82. doi:10.1186/s13063-016-1206-7

McDermott, R., Campbell, S., Li, M., & McCulloch, B. (2009). The health and nutrition of young Indigenous women in north Queensland—intergenerational implications of poor food quality, obesity, diabetes, tobacco smoking and alcohol use. *Public Health Nutrition*, *12*(11), 2143-2149.

McMurray, A., & Clendon, J. (2015). *Community health and wellness. Primary health care in practice* (5th ed.). Chatswood: Elsevier.

Moore, T. (2015). *Engaging and partnering with vulnerable families and communities: The keys to effective place-based approaches*. Goulburn Child FIRST Alliance Conference 2015—The NEXT Generation: The future of our children and young people's safety is in our hands.

Moore, T.G., McDonald, M., Sanjeevan, S., & Price, A. (2012). *Sustained home visiting for vulnerable families and children: A literature review of effective processes and strategies*. Parkville: Centre for Community Child Health, Royal Children's Hospital. Retrieved from http://www.rch.org.au/uploadedFiles/Main/Content/ccch/resources_and_publications/Home_visiting_ lit_review_RAH_processes_final.pdf

Moore, T. G., Arefadib, N., Deery, A., Keyes, M., & West, S. (2017). *The first thousand days: An evidence paper—Summary*. Parkville: Centre for Community Child Health, Murdoch Children's Research Institute. Retrieved from http://royalfarwest.org.au/wp-content/uploads/2017/12/Murdoch-Report.pdf

Moss, B., Harper, H., & Silburn, S. (2015). Strengthening Aboriginal child development in central Australia through a universal preschool readiness program. *Australasian Journal of Early Childhood*, *40*(4), 13-20.

Munns, A., & Walker, R. (2015). The Halls Creek community families program: Elements of role of the child health nurse in development of a remote Aboriginal home visiting peer support program for families in the early years. *Australian Journal of Rural Health*, *23*, 322-326

Munns, A., Toye, C., Hegney, D., Kickett, M., Marriott, R., & Walker, R. (2018). Aboriginal parent support: A partnership approach. *Journal of Clinical Nursing*, 27, e437-e450. doi:10.1111/jocn.13979

Mutch, R. C., Watkins, R., & Bower, C. (2015). Fetal alcohol spectrum disorders: Notifications to the Western Australian Register of Developmental Anomalies. *Journal of Paediatrics and Child Health*, *51*, 433-443.

National Aboriginal Health Strategy Working Party. (1989). *National Aboriginal health strategy*. Canberra: Author.

National Health and Medical Research Council. (2012). *Infant feeding guidelines. Information for health workers*. Canberra: Author. Retrieved from https://www.nhmrc.gov.au/_files_nhmrc/file/publications/170131_n56_infant_feeding_guidelines.pdf

Nicholson, J. M., Lucas, N., Berthelsen, D., & Wake, M. (2012). Socioeconomic inequality profiles in physical and developmental health from 0-7 years: Australian National Study. *Journal of Epidemiology & Community Health*, *66*, 81-87.

Ou, L., Chen, J., Garrett, P., & Hillman, K. (2010). Ethnic and Indigenous access to early childhood healthcare services in Australia: Parents' perceived unmet needs and related barriers. *Australian and New Zealand Journal of Public Health*, *35*: 30-37.

O'Leary, C. M., Halliday, J., Bartu, A., D'Antoine, H., & Bower, C. (2013). Alcohol-use disorders during and within one year of pregnancy: A population-based cohort study 1985–2006. *BJOG*, *120*(6), 744-753.

Pillas, D., Marmot, M., Naicker, K., Goldblatt, P., Morrison, J., & Pilkhart, H. (2014). Social inequalities in early childhood health and development: A European-wide systematic review. *Pediatr Res*, *76*, 418-424.

Ritte, R., Panozzo, S., Johnston, L., Agerholm, J., Kvernmo, S. E., Rowely, K., & Arabena, K. (2016). An Australian model of the first 1000 days: An Indigenous-led process to turn an international initiative into an early-life strategy benefiting in indigenous families. *Global health, Epidemiology and Genomics*, *1*(e11), 1-10. doi:10.1017/gheg.2016.7

Royal Children's Hospital. (n.d.). *Impetigo (school sores)*. Retrieved from https://www.rch.org.au/kidsinfo/fact_sheets/impetigo_school_sores

Rumbold, A. R., & Cunningham, J. (2008). A review of the impact of antenatal care for Australian Indigenous women and attempts to strengthen these services. *Maternal and Child Health Journal*, *12*(1), 83-100. doi:10.1007/s10995-007-0216-1

Sayers, S., & Boyle, J. (2010). Indigenous perinatal and neonatal outcomes: A time for prevention strategies. *Journal of Paediatric Child Health*, *46*, 475-478.

Schultz, C., Walker, R., Bessarab, D., McMillan, F., Macleod, J., & Marriott, R. (2014). Interdisciplinary care to enhance mental health and social and emotional wellbeing.

In P. Dudgeon, H. Milroy & R. Walker (Eds.), *Working together: Aboriginal and Torres Strait Islander mental health and wellbeing principles and practice* (2nd ed., pp. 221-242). Canberra: Department of the Prime Minister and Cabinet.

Shonkoff, J. P., & Garner, A. S. (2012).The lifelong effects of early childhood adversity and toxic stress. *Pediatrics*, *129*, 232-246.

Simpson, S., D'Aprano, A., Tayler, C., Toon Khoo, S., & Highfold, R. (2016). Validation of a culturally adapted developmental screening tool for Australian Aboriginal children: Early findings and next steps. *Early Human Development*, *103*, 91-95.

Steenkamp, M., Boyle, J., Kildea, S., Moore, V., Davies, M., & Rumbold, A. (2017). Perinatal outcomes among young Indigenous Australian mothers: A cross-sectional study and comparison with adult Indigenous mothers. *Birth*, *44*, 262-271. https://doi.org/10.1111/birt.12283

Taylor, K., & Guerin, P. (2014). *Health care and Indigenous Australians. Cultural safety in practice*. South Yarra: Palgrave.

Webb, R., & Wilson, N. (2013). Rheumatic fever in New Zealand. *Journal of Paediatric Child Health*, *49*, 179-184.

Weetra, D., Glover, K., Buckskin, M., Kit, J. A., Leane, C., Mitchell, A., ... Brown S. J. (2016). Stressful events, social health issues and psychological distress in Aboriginal women having a baby in South Australia: Implications for antenatal care. *BMC Pregnancy and Childbirth*, *16*, 88.

Wise, S. (2013). *Improving the early life outcomes of Indigenous children: Implementing early childhood development at a local level*. Issues paper no. 6. Produced for Closing the Gap Clearinghouse. Canberra: Australian Institute of Health and Welfare & Melbourne: Australian Institute of Family Studies.

Wong, R., Herceg, A., Patterson, C., Freebairn, L., Baker, A., Sharp, P., ... Tongs, J. (2011). Positive impact of a long-running urban Aboriginal medical service midwifery program. *Aust N Z J Obstet Gynaecol*, *51*(6), 518-522.

World Health Organization. (2011). *Exclusive breastfeeding for six months best for babies everywhere*. Retrieved from http://www.who.int/mediacentre/news/statements/2011/breastfeeding_20110115/en

World Health Organization. (2019). *Trachoma*. Retrieved from https://www.who.int/newsroom/fact-sheets/detail/trachoma

Zubrick, S. R., Shepherd, C., Dudgeon, P., Gee, G., Paradies, Y., Scrine, C., & Walker, R. (2014). Social determinants of social and emotional wellbeing. In P. Dudgeon, H. Milroy & R. Walker (Eds.), *Working together: Aboriginal and Torres Strait Islander mental health and wellbeing principles and practice* (2nd ed., pp. 93-112). Canberra: Department of the Prime Minister and Cabinet.

CHAPTER **EIGHT**

Mental health and social and emotional wellbeing

Faye McMillan, Thomas Brideson and Sally Drummond

LEARNING CONCEPTS

Studying this chapter should enable you to learn about mental health in the contemporary Australian environment through the following:

1. bring context to current mental health in Australia.
2. become aware of Aboriginal and Torres Strait Islander leadership in the mental health space through the *Gayaa Dhuwi (Proud Spirit) Declaration*.
3. determine future directions for Aboriginal and Torres Strait Islander peoples' mental health.
4. explore the role of the healthcare professional in Aboriginal and Torres Strait Islander peoples' mental health.
5. understand mental health workforce development.

KEY TERMS

Fifth National Mental Health and Suicide Prevention Plan

Gayaa Dhuwi (Proud Spirit) Declaration

mental health

National Strategic Framework for Aboriginal and Torres Strait Islander Peoples' Mental Health and Social and Emotional Wellbeing 2017–2023

social and emotional wellbeing

suicide prevention

United Nations Declaration on the Rights of Indigenous Peoples

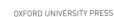

Introduction

social and emotional wellbeing A term used to describe the social, emotional, spiritual and cultural wellbeing of a person. It recognises that connection to land, culture, spirituality, family and community can influence wellbeing, and recognises that a person's social and emotional wellbeing is influenced by past and current policies and events.

Aboriginal and Torres Strait Islander peoples experience poorer health and **social and emotional wellbeing** outcomes over the lifespan than non-Indigenous Australians; for example, Aboriginal and Torres Strait Islander adults experience higher rates of psychological distress, and youth experience higher rates of intentional self-harm (Dudgeon, Walker, Scrine, Shepherd, Calma & Ring, 2014). The way Aboriginal and Torres Strait Islander peoples view mental health and social and emotional wellbeing is unlike the view of non-Indigenous Australians, and has been affected by and affects prevention and intervention initiatives and the policies that underpin these initiatives.

Evidence suggests that programs with a holistic, trauma-informed recovery focus are more likely to be successful than the short-term, inflexible, one-shoe-fits-all approach of the past. Importantly, policies that encourage trauma-informed practice are vital in shaping the delivery of healthcare, as discussed in the second part of this chapter.

Aboriginal and Torres Strait Islander peoples' mental health: a national priority

suicide prevention A commitment to reduce the risk of an individual taking their own life.

Fifth National Mental Health and Suicide Prevention Plan A commitment from all governments to work together to achieve integrated planning and service delivery of mental health and suicide prevention related services.

In October 2017, Aboriginal and Torres Strait Islander peoples' mental health and **suicide prevention** became a national priority for the first time. Priority area 4 of the **Fifth National Mental Health and Suicide Prevention Plan** (the Fifth Plan) is: 'Improving Aboriginal and Torres Strait Islander mental health and suicide prevention' (Australian Government, 2017a, p. 30). The plan was endorsed by the Council of Australian Governments (COAG), which comprises the Commonwealth Government and all state and territory governments within Australia. While the priority is to be welcomed, all people involved in mental health and human services need to be mindful that all the other priority areas relate to Aboriginal and Torres Strait Islander peoples and therefore consideration of these is also required. This is articulated in the Implementation Plan of the *Fifth National Mental Health and Suicide Prevention Plan* (Australian Government, 2017a, p. 49).

There has been strong advocacy for priority area 4 over many years and it is a welcomed inclusion into the Fifth Plan. Advocacy dates back to the late 1980s with the National Aboriginal Health Strategy (National Aboriginal Health Strategy Working Party, 1989) and throughout the 1990s through the national consultancy report, *Ways Forward* (Swan & Raphael, 1995), the 1995 article 'Aboriginal and Torres Strait Islander Mental Health and Social and Emotional Wellbeing' (Calma, Dudgeon & Bray,

2017) and the *Bringing Them Home* report (Wilson & Australian Human Rights and Equal Opportunity Commission, 1997). Further advocacy took place with the *National Strategic Framework for Aboriginal and Torres Strait Islander Peoples' Mental Health and Social and Emotional Well Being 2004–2009* (Social Health Reference Group, 2004).

Since the signing of the Statement of Intent that emerged from the Close the Gap Campaign, there has been an increased effort to focus attention on **mental health** and suicide prevention for Aboriginal and Torres Strait Islander peoples. Among many developments there has been the release of the *National Aboriginal and Torres Strait Islander Suicide Prevention Strategy* (Australian Government, 2013), the launch of the *Gayaa Dhuwi (Proud Spirit) Declaration* (National Aboriginal and Torres Strait Islander Leadership in Mental Health, 2015a) and the revised **National Strategic Framework for Aboriginal and Torres Strait Islander Peoples' Mental Health and Social and Emotional Wellbeing 2017–2023** (Australian Government, 2017b). These three documents are referred to in the Fifth Plan, which commits all governments and agencies to the implementation of the *Gayaa Dhuwi (Proud Spirit) Declaration*. It also commits all governments and agencies to the *National Strategic Framework for Aboriginal and Torres Strait Islander Peoples' Mental Health and Social and Emotional Well Being 2004–2009* to guide all activity in this priority.

mental health 'A state of wellbeing in which every individual realises his or her own potential, can cope with the normal stresses of life, can work productively and fruitfully, and is able to make a contribution to her or his community' (World Health Organization, 2014).

National Strategic Framework for Aboriginal and Torres Strait Islander Peoples' Mental Health and Social and Emotional Wellbeing 2017–2023 A framework dedicated to Aboriginal and Torres Strait Islander peoples' social and emotional wellbeing and mental health.

Gayaa Dhuwi (Proud Spirit) Declaration

Launched in 2015, the **Gayaa Dhuwi (Proud Spirit) Declaration** was developed by the National Aboriginal and Torres Strait Islander Leadership in Mental Health. The *Gayaa Dhuwi (Proud Spirit) Declaration* describes the critical need for Aboriginal and Torres Strait Islander leadership across all parts of the Australian mental health system to achieve the highest attainable standard of mental health and suicide prevention outcomes for Aboriginal and Torres Strait Islander peoples. In a media release at the time of the launch, Tom Calma stated:

Gayaa Dhuwi (Proud Spirit) Declaration A commitment to improve the mental health of Aboriginal and Torres Strait Islander peoples. The name of the declaration was coined from 'Gayaa', which means happy, pleased and proud, and 'Dhuwi', which means 'spirit' in the Yuwaalaraay and Gamilaraay languages of northwest New South Wales.

> It's time for action if the mental health of our peoples is to improve, and for our suicide rates to come down to at least the same as that of other Australians. We must cement Indigenous leadership as fundamental and non-negotiable in that response, and the *Gayaa Dhuwi (Proud Spirit) Declaration* provides framework [sic] for that.
>
> National Aboriginal and Torres Strait Islander Leadership in Mental Health (2015b, p. 2)

The five themes of the *Gayaa Dhuwi (Proud Spirit) Declaration* are:

1. Aboriginal and Torres Strait Islander concepts of social and emotional wellbeing, mental health and healing should be recognised across all parts of the Australian mental health system, and in some circumstances support specialised areas of practice.

2. Aboriginal and Torres Strait Islander concepts of social and emotional wellbeing, mental health and healing combined with clinical perspectives will make the greatest contribution to the achievement of the highest attainable standard of mental health and suicide prevention outcomes for Aboriginal and Torres Strait Islander peoples.

3. Aboriginal and Torres Strait Islander values-based social and emotional wellbeing and mental health outcome measures in combination with clinical outcome measures should guide the assessment of mental health and suicide prevention services and programs for Aboriginal and Torres Strait Islander peoples.

4. Aboriginal and Torres Strait Islander presence and leadership is required across all parts of the Australian mental health system for it to adapt to, and be accountable to, Aboriginal and Torres Strait Islander peoples for the achievement of the highest attainable standard of mental health and suicide prevention outcomes.

5. Aboriginal and Torres Strait Islander leaders should be supported and valued to be visible and influential across all parts of the Australian mental health system.

National Aboriginal and Torres Strait Islander Leadership in Mental Health
(2015b, pp. 4–5)

Under each of these themes are a number of actions required to meet the needs of the declaration. Of particular relevance to this chapter are the following actions:

2.2 It is the responsibility of all mental health professionals and professional associations, and educational institutions and standard-setting bodies that work in mental health (and also those in areas related to mental health, particularly suicide prevention) to make their practices and/or curriculum respectful and inclusive of the mental health and suicide prevention needs of Aboriginal and Torres Strait Islander peoples, as outlined in this Declaration.

National Aboriginal and Torres Strait Islander Leadership in Mental Health
(2015b, p. 4)

4.1 Aboriginal and Torres Strait Islander people should be trained, employed, empowered and valued to work at all levels and across all parts of the Australian mental health system and among the professions that work in that system.

National Aboriginal and Torres Strait Islander Leadership in Mental Health
(2015b, p. 5)

The essence of these actions is targeting the responsibilities of the professions in mental health and human services to ensure they increase their efforts to respond to mental health needs of Aboriginal and Torres Strait Islander peoples. These calls have been made over decades and they require restating as we have yet to have this responsibility of workforce development fully realised. There remain limited long-term effective strategies dedicated to increase the numbers of this workforce by the major professions in mental health or to make these professions accountable to the multitude of documents stating this need over decades. This call has been made by Aboriginal and Torres Strait Islander peoples since the 1970s and Aboriginal and Torres Strait Islander peoples continue to wait for these responsibilities and professional parity. This responsibility remains an issue for the professions to roll up their sleeves and seek ways of working with Aboriginal and Torres Strait Islander peoples on effectively delivering suitable arrangements of program delivery and flexibility. What we do know is that saying and doing are not the same thing, and have not resulted in the desired outcome.

The *Gayaa Dhuwi (Proud Spirit) Declaration* is listed for implementation in the *Fifth National Mental Health and Suicide Prevention Plan*. Since the release of the Fifth Plan, National Aboriginal and Torres Strait Islander Leadership in Mental Health developed and launched *Gayaa Dhuwi (Proud Spirit) Declaration Implementation Guide* (2018a) and *Health in Culture—Policy Concordance* (2018b) on Close the Gap Day, 15 March 2018.

Gayaa Dhuwi (Proud Spirit) Declaration Implementation Guide provides a comprehensive guide for governments and organisations across the mental health system to implementing the *Gayaa Dhuwi (Proud Spirit) Declaration* as per Article 12.3 of the *Fifth National Mental Health and Suicide Prevention Plan*.

Health in Culture—Policy Concordance (National Aboriginal and Torres Strait Islander Leadership in Mental Health, 2018b) cross-references documents as diverse as the *Fifth National Mental Health and Suicide Prevention Plan*, the *National Strategic Framework for Aboriginal and Torres Strait Islander Peoples' Mental Health and Social and Emotional Wellbeing 2017–2023*, the *National Aboriginal and Torres Strait Islander Health Plan 2013–2023* (Commonwealth of Australia, 2013) and the *Gayaa Dhuwi (Proud Spirit) Declaration*, among many others. It sets out clearly what is required of Australian governments, primary healthcare networks and the mental health system overall to improve the social and emotional wellbeing and mental health of, and prevent suicide among, Aboriginal and Torres Strait Islander peoples.

United Nations Declaration on the Rights of Indigenous Peoples

On 13 September 2007, The **United Nations Declaration on the Rights of Indigenous Peoples (UNDRIP)** was adopted by the General Assembly of the United Nations. This historic document 'establishes a universal framework of minimum standards for the survival, dignity and well-being of the indigenous peoples of the world and it elaborates on existing human rights standards and fundamental freedoms as they apply to the specific situation of indigenous peoples' (United Nations, 2008, para. 2). The Declaration is a significant leap forward in the recognition, promotion and protection of the rights and freedoms of indigenous peoples.

United Nations Declaration on the Rights of Indigenous Peoples A framework of minimum standards for the survival, dignity, wellbeing and rights of the world's indigenous peoples.

In 2014, as a result of this document and the successful partnership that forged it, the United Nations held the first World Conference on Indigenous Peoples. This resulted in a commitment to the UNDRIP, the start of many collaborations.

Future directions for Aboriginal and Torres Strait Islander peoples' mental health

The National Strategic Framework for Aboriginal and Torres Strait Islander Peoples' Mental Health and Social and Emotional Wellbeing 2017–2023 (Australian Government, 2017b) is listed as guiding activity within the *Fifth National Mental Health and Suicide Prevention Plan*. The vision of the Framework is

> [for] Aboriginal and Torres Strait Islander people, families and communities to achieve and sustain the highest attainable standard of social and emotional wellbeing and mental health supported by mental health and related services that are effective, high quality, clinically and culturally appropriate, and affordable.
>
> Australian Government (2017b, p. 27)

The Framework articulates strengthening the foundations as key to improvements, identifying three key areas to do so: an effective and empowered workforce, a strong evidence base and effective partnerships.

Significant key strategies listed within the Framework include the need for particular attention on emerging Aboriginal and Torres Strait Islander mental health workforces and developing appropriate career pathways, support and professional standing for them. These emerging workforces have emerged due to the professions not building an effective set of strategies to increase their own numbers to a level of parity.

Psychological trauma

This section will discuss psychological trauma, including the definitions commonly cited, and provide detail of trauma-informed care. These are important concepts in relation to intergenerational trauma experienced by Aboriginal and Torres Strait Islander peoples.

Trauma is a word commonly used in our everyday language and means different things to different health professionals. Ask health professionals working within an emergency department what 'trauma' is and they will likely speak about physical trauma as a result of injury sustained to the body. When asking the same question to health professionals working within the human services or mental health sectors, they will likely speak about psychological injury and such concepts as developmental and complex trauma.

Within the psychological context, trauma is defined as occurring when an individual's internal and external resources are insufficient to manage an external threat (real or perceived); it can arise from a single event or multiple and/or sustained experiences (Terr, 1990). Traumatic events happen to all people, across all ages and groups. However, psychological trauma and its consequences are not specific to the event in question, but rather to the individual's experience of the event and response or responses to it, meaning not all individuals will experience or respond to an event or events in the same way (Van der Kolk & McFarlane, 1996).

Definitions of types of psychological trauma

As discussed, psychological trauma presents in many different forms, depending on the circumstances and the personalities and life experiences of the people involved. Common forms include the following:

- *Complex trauma*—the experiencing of numerous traumatic events that are frequently invasive and interpersonal in nature, and can include severe and pervasive abuse and neglect (Atkinson, 2012).
- *Developmental trauma*—childhood trauma that occurs in the first years of life. This type of trauma can affect the brain's ability to develop in a normal growth sequence. This has been identified as the single most important health challenge of our time (van der Kolk, 2007).
- *Generational trauma*—the concept of unresolved trauma from one generation being passed on to future generations, resulting in a normalisation of the associated behaviours (Atkinson, 2012).
- *Collective or social trauma*—trauma resulting from a shared traumatic experience by a group of people, including whole social groups. This type of trauma can comprise a collective or shared traumatic memory (Atkinson, 2012).
- *Historical–cultural trauma*—a shared experience and memory of events in the mind of the individual and/or community, passed throughout the generations (Atkinson, 2012).
- *Vicarious trauma*—trauma that affects a person who did not directly experience the trauma, but is close to or professionally assisting the person who did. It can be accumulative, and the greater the exposure to traumatic material, the greater the risk of trauma (Kezelman & Stavropoulos, 2018).

Effects of trauma

Individuals all respond differently to experiences of trauma. Although both adults and children may experience trauma, when a child experiences developmental trauma the effect on the developing brain can be profound. Trauma can create consequences for the individual such as a loss of safety and connection, fear, helplessness, powerlessness, self-destructive and other destructive behaviours, and poorer overall health outcomes (Kezelman & Stavropoulos, 2018).

The experience of trauma can bring about responses that are commonly known as 'survival responses' within the body. These responses are automatic and operate outside our conscious awareness; for example, the person may become hyper-aroused or disengaged. If an initial trauma is not resolved, this survival response can continue to be a trigger and the survival responses can be activated by minor stressors (Kezelman & Stavropoulos, 2018).

A trauma-informed approach

Trauma-informed practice is based on the foundation that survivors of trauma have specific vulnerabilities that may be triggered in some circumstances or situations (Kezelman & Stavropoulos, 2012). Trauma-informed practice is a strengths-based framework, founded on six fundamental principles—safety, trustworthiness, choice, collaboration, empowerment and respect for diversity—with the first principle of the health professional or service provider being to do no further harm. Trauma-informed services embody a culture of not re-traumatising or blaming victims for their traumatic reactions, but of understanding that with hope and optimism recovery is possible for the unique individuals who have experienced these events and have managed as best as they were able (Kezelman & Stavropoulos, 2012).

Case study 8.1

A multi-generational family's story

This case study uses a multi-generational family approach to explore the mental health and social and emotional wellbeing concerns that can manifest across and through generations. This case study will be utilised to provide a greater understanding of the impact of past policies and practices on families and individuals.

As health professionals we can often overlook the persuasive nature of circumstances and events that have shaped families and individuals when presenting for healthcare. Depending on the presentation, these events can significantly influence engagement and health outcomes.

Sarah (born in the 1990s): daughter of Cindy, granddaughter of Leslie and great-granddaughter of Nan

Perinatal mental health—attachment
Sarah is a 27-year-old woman with two children aged six months and two years. Sarah is separated from the father of her children and has recently moved back

to her childhood home with her parents to support her through this difficult time. Sarah and her children do not have any contact at present with the father or the paternal side of the children's family. Sarah is a nurse and has enrolled in university to study midwifery, but has taken a leave of absence due to the stress of the separation and being the sole carer for two infant children.

Cindy (born in the 1970s): granddaughter of Nan, daughter of Leslie and mother of Sarah

Experienced trauma—insecure attachment with mother
Cindy is a 50-year-old woman. A local preschool teacher, she has been married for 28 years to her husband of the same age. Cindy has a good relationship for the most part with her mother, Leslie. Although Cindy did not have an easy childhood, and experienced significant trauma and an insecure attachment to her mother, she feels that the positives and negatives of her own experience of being a child have helped her to become the parent she is today, allowing her to make decisions in regards to her life that fostered strong and stable attachments. These included her drive to become a tertiary educated mature-age student, to assist in secure employment and to role-model the importance of education to her children.

Leslie: born in the 1940s, daughter of Nan, mother of Cindy and grandmother of Sarah

Post-traumatic stress disorder; poor parenting role model due to role modelling—attachment.
Leslie is 70 years old and is originally from Queensland. Leslie was a stay-at-home mother who lived with her husband and has five adult children, of which only one lives locally (Cindy, the youngest), offering regular in-person contact. Leslie was removed from her mother's care when she was an infant and although she had sporadic contact with her mother throughout her childhood, she grew up predominantly in a girls' home. The home was five hours away from her family home and was 'off country'. After finishing school she went to work for a local family as a housekeeper, where she met her husband-to-be, a local Aboriginal farm hand who had grown up with his biological parents off country. Leslie's husband died in a work accident while she was pregnant with her last child Cindy. Leslie did not get the chance to tell her husband she was pregnant prior to his death.

After this significant loss, Leslie became disconnected from her husband's family, and felt a great sense of loss—of her husband, partner and main support, and of his family. It was at this time that Leslie acutely felt a sense of not belonging to the country and being a stranger on the land she lived. As a

(Continued)

result, Leslie set out to reconnect with her family and country, only to find out that her biological parents and grandparents had all passed away and that all known siblings were scattered across the country with no reliable information about their names or how to contact them. Although Leslie had solid group of friends from her time in the girls' home, her contact with them is now sporadic.

The feeling of being alone in the world, coupled with insecure attachments and a lack of functional role models during her own childhood have impacted on Leslie's ability to form secure attachments with her own children, resulting in the children—particularly Cindy—becoming parentified from an early age. This dependence on Cindy has only increased as she has aged. Throughout her adult life she has experienced episodic depression, which at times was treated with medication, but she has never really engaged in counselling due to trust issues with government and other agencies, as well as the stigma of having a mental health issue.

Nan: born in the 1920s, now deceased, mother of Leslie, grandmother of Cindy and great-grandmother of Sarah

During Nan's time as a parent, children were moved around within their kinship family to share responsibility and care, and to keep the children safe, due to the impact of government policies at the time. Nan at times felt that she was a terrible parent and felt guilty when her children were in the care of other family members, and this guilt was often coupled with bouts of anxiety for the safety of the children. However, when the children were in her care she was often challenged with regards to parenting, being hyper-vigilant and displaying high levels of emotional distress. This was exacerbated when members of the Aborigines Protection Board arrived in her community, with the ever-present threat of forcibly removing children from their families, meaning she had to send her children to other family members on short notice.

Leslie's presentation

During a community RUOK day, Leslie is talking to a health professional staffing the community health stand. During the conversation, Leslie appears agitated (constantly wringing her hands and moving her lower extremities) and describes her poor sleep pattern with associated nightmares and being teary for no apparent reason. During the discussion, Leslie states that she is very distressed by events depicted on the news of children being forcibly removed from their parents in other countries. Leslie goes on to say that she is worried about the impact of her granddaughter Sarah's separation from the father of her children. The health professional is known to Leslie and has a good relationship with the family.

You are the health professional staffing the stand. What would be your next step in supporting Leslie in seeking appropriate healthcare support for her concerns? Consider the scope of your own professional practice in deciding what would be the most appropriate course of action for you to take. In your considerations, identify your role as the professional and possible ethical issues such as confidentiality and dual relationships that often exist when working with individuals and families.

CRITICAL REFLECTION QUESTIONS

- What policies of the day would have impacted on the people in the case study?
- What do you perceive as your professional role within the mental health space?
- What are the key considerations that arise for Leslie's mental health?
- What is your professional response within your scope of practice to Leslie's mental health concerns?
- What might be ethical considerations within the presenting case study of Leslie?

Case study 8.2

Sarah's story

After being referred by her GP, Sarah presents to the local mental health service with anxiety symptoms. She says these have been present for her 'whole life' but have been harder to control in the last year, and they 'have gotten much worse' when she began her HSC year at school. Sarah describes that she is consistently 'worried' about things. She is concerned that the worry is getting harder to dismiss and would like some strategies to help manage her worries. Sarah's GP has ruled out any medical causes for her presentation.

Sarah grew up in inner-city Sydney, which she loved. She reports she was a 'bright and happy' child, but recalls worrying about things like school, making friends, staying over at friends' houses, and the health of her family. She reports excelling in school and extracurricular activities, and was advanced in meeting her developmental milestones.

Sarah is the eldest of three children, and now lives with her mother and father in a small rural town after Sarah's mother was relocated for work. Sarah is now completing her final year at a new school. Sarah's teachers have expressed their concern that her school performance is deteriorating, that she is not

(Continued)

paying attention in class, and that she is not getting her work in on time. Sarah reports she is constantly worried about everything, including making decisions.

Sarah reports no symptoms consistent with delusions, hallucinations or disorganised thinking, or anything that would indicate the presence of mania. A risk assessment reveals that Sarah has no significant past history of risk and no recent thoughts, plans or symptoms suggesting risk: no self-harm, past or present, no risk identified with regards to harm to others, and no suicidal ideation, past or present.

CRITICAL REFLECTION QUESTIONS

- What social and emotional wellbeing concerns are present in this case study?
- What is your role as a health professional in providing person-centred care for Sarah?
- What are the key considerations that arise for Sarah's mental health?
- Within your scope of practice, what is your professional response to Sarah's mental health concerns?
- What might be ethical considerations within the presenting case study of Sarah? Consider her age.

IMPLICATIONS FOR NURSING AND ALLIED HEALTH PRACTICE

In the Australian context, with mental health being a national priority, a multi-faceted and multi-disciplinary approach is the responsibility of the entire health workforce. This includes a greater undergraduate focus on mental health and social and emotional wellbeing within health disciplines, with respect to the roles and responsibilities of nursing and allied health professions. As part of their professional development, every individual requires an appreciation and working knowledge of their impact on the mental wellness of individuals and communities. This chapter has highlighted the important need for an appropriately trained and skilled mental health workforce for working with Aboriginal and Torres Strait Islander communities and individuals to reduce the impact and incidence of mental ill health.

CRITICAL-REFLECTION QUESTIONS

- What factors may impact your own mental health and social and emotional wellbeing? (Remember you are a whole person, so your answer should be reflective of your personal and professional spheres.)

- Are you able to identify strategies that either have enhanced or continue to enhance your own mental health?
- What is your understanding of unconscious bias, and how might this impact your daily life?
- What is your understanding of professional bias, and how might this impact professional relationships?

Conclusion

This chapter has introduced a number of documents that support and influence the continued development of a mental health workforce that elevates and supports Aboriginal and Torres Strait Islander peoples' histories and lived experiences in the establishment of equitable services to meet their holistic and person-centred health needs. These include the *Fifth National Mental Health and Suicide Prevention Plan*, the *Gayaa Dhuwi (Proud Spirit) Declaration* and the United Nations Declaration on the Rights of Indigenous Peoples. These are important concepts and documents, particularly in relation to intergenerational trauma that is experienced in Aboriginal and Torres Strait Islander communities. Trauma and trauma-informed practice are integral to the holistic practice of the nurse and allied health professional.

SUMMARY

Learning concept 1

Bring context to current mental health practices in Australia: Mental health and social and emotional wellbeing continues to be a priority within the Australian context. Mental health is everybody's responsibility and influences every aspect of human life, inclusive of our personal and professional lives. It is your responsibility to ensure evidenced-based and culturally appropriate mental healthcare for all individuals and communities you interact with.

Learning concept 2

Become aware of Aboriginal and Torres Strait Islander leadership in the mental health space through the *Gayaa Dhuwi (Proud Spirit) Declaration*: The Declaration describes the critical need for Aboriginal and Torres Strait Islander leadership across all parts of the Australian mental health system to achieve the highest attainable standard of mental health and suicide prevention outcomes for Aboriginal and Torres Strait Islander peoples.

Learning concept 3

Determine future directions for Aboriginal and Torres Strait Islander peoples' mental health: Future directions are underpinned by the *National Strategic Framework for Aboriginal and Torres Strait Islander Peoples' Mental Health and Social and Emotional Wellbeing 2017–2023*.

Learning concept 4

Explore the role of the healthcare professional in Aboriginal and Torres Strait Islander peoples' mental health: With mental health being a national priority, the role of the healthcare professional is fundamental. A multi-faceted and multi-disciplinary approach is the responsibility of the entire health workforce.

Learning concept 5

Understand mental health workforce development: There is a pressing need for appropriately trained and skilled mental health professionals working with Aboriginal and Torres Strait Islander communities and individuals to reduce the impact and incidence of mental ill health.

REVISION QUESTIONS

1. What is the significance of the *Fifth National Mental Health and Suicide Prevention Plan* for Aboriginal and Torres Strait Islander peoples?
2. What do you see as the important contribution that the *Gayaa Dhuwi (Proud Spirit) Declaration* makes to the mental health space in Australia?
3. Can you define and describe your role as a health professional as it applies to working with individuals and communities with mental health concerns?
4. How is your own mental health and what proactive measures are you able to take to sustain and enhance your own mental health?

FURTHER READINGS/ADDITIONAL RESOURCES

Australian Institute of Health and Welfare: http://www.aihw.gov.au

National Aboriginal and Torres Strait Islander Leadership in Mental Health: http://natsilmh. org.au/resources

United Nations Declaration on the Rights of Indigenous Peoples: https://www.un.org/ development/desa/indigenouspeoples/declaration-on-the-rights-of-indigenous-peoples.html

REFERENCES

Atkinson, J. (2012). *Educating a trauma informed approach to healing generational trauma for Aboriginal Australians*. Retrieved from http://www.fwtdp.org.au/wp-content/uploads/2013/08/Judy-Atkinson-Healing-From-Generational-Trauma-Workbook.pdf

Australia. National Aboriginal Health Strategy Working Party. (1989). *A national Aboriginal health strategy*. Canberra: National Aboriginal Health Strategy Working Party.

Australian Government. (2013). National Aboriginal and Torres Strait Islander suicide prevention strategy. Canberra: Department of Health and Ageing. Retrieved from http://www.health.gov.au/internet/main/publishing.nsf/content/mental-pub-atsi-suicide-prevention-strategy

Australian Government. (2017a). *The Fifth National Mental Health and Suicide Prevention Plan*. Canberra: Department of Health. Retrieved from http://www.coaghealthcouncil.gov.au/Portals/0/Fifth%20National%20Mental%20Health%20and%20Suicide%20Prevention%20Plan.pdf

Australian Government. (2017b). *National Strategic Framework for Aboriginal and Torres Strait Islander Peoples' Mental Health and Social and Emotional Wellbeing 2017-2023*. Canberra: Department of the Prime Minister and Cabinet. Retrieved from https://www.pmc.gov.au/resource-centre/indigenous-affairs/national-strategic-framework-mental-health-social-emotional-wellbeing-2017-23

Calma, T., Dudgeon, P., & Bray, A. (2017). Aboriginal and Torres Strait Islander Social and Emotional Wellbeing and Mental Health. *Australian Psychologist*, *52*(4), 255-260. doi:10.1111/ap.12299

Commonwealth of Australia. (2013). *National Aboriginal and Torres Strait Islander Health Plan 2013–2023*, Commonwealth of Australia: Canberra.

Dudgeon, P., Walker, R., Scrine, C., Shepherd, C., Calma, T., & Ring, I. (2014). *Effective strategies to strengthen the mental health and wellbeing of Aboriginal and Torres Strait Islander people*. Issues paper no. 12. Closing the Gap Clearinghouse. AIHW/AIFS.

Kezelman, C. A., & Stavropoulos, P. A. (2012). *Practice guidelines for treatment of complex trauma and trauma informed care and service delivery*. Kirribilli: Adults Surviving Child Abuse. Retrieved from https://www.recoveryonpurpose.com/upload/ASCA_Practice%20Guidelines%20for%20the%20Treatment%20of%20Complex%20Trauma.pdf

Kezelman, C. A., & Stavropoulos, P. A. (2018). *Talking about trauma: Guide to conversations and screening for health and other service providers*. Blue Knot Foundation. Retrieved from https://www.blueknot.org.au/Portals/2/Newsletter/Talking%20About%20Trauma%20Services_WEB.pdf?ver=2018-04-06-160830-113

National Aboriginal Health Strategy Working Party. (1989). *A national Aboriginal health strategy*. Canberra: National Aboriginal Health Strategy Working Party

National Aboriginal and Torres Strait Islander Leadership in Mental Health. (2015a). *Gayaa Dhuwi (Proud Spirit) Declaration*. NATSILMH. Retrieved from http://natsilmh.org.au/sites/default/files/gayaa_dhuwi_declaration_A4.pdf

National Aboriginal and Torres Strait Islander Leadership in Mental Health. (2015b). *Indigenous leadership needed to address mental health crisis* [Media release], 27 August.

Retrieved from http://natsilmh.org.au/sites/default/files/Gayaa%20Dhuwi%20Media%20 Release_Final.pdf

National Aboriginal and Torres Strait Islander Leadership in Mental Health. (2018a). *Gayaa Dhuwi (Proud Spirit) Declaration Implementation Guide*. NATSILMH. Retrieved from http://natsilmh.org.au/sites/default/files/Health%20in%20Culture%20GDD%20 Implementation%20Guide.pdf

National Aboriginal and Torres Strait Islander Leadership in Mental Health. (2018b). *Health in culture—policy concordance*. NATSILMH. Retrieved from http://natsilmh.org.au/sites/ default/files/NATSILMH%20Health%20in%20Culture%20Policy%20Concordance%20 %282%29.pdf

Social Health Reference Group. (2004). *National strategic framework for Aboriginal and Torres Strait Islander peoples' mental health and social and emotional well being, 2004–2009*. National Aboriginal and Torres Strait Islander Health Council and National Mental Health Working Group. Retrieved from https://www.ahmrc.org.au/media/resources/social-emotional-wellbeing/mental-health/328-national-strategic-framework-for-aboriginal-and-torres-strait-islander-peoples-mental-health-and-social-and-emotional-well-being-2004-2009/file.html

Swan, P., & Raphael, B. (1995). *Ways forward. National consultancy report on Aboriginal and Torres Strait Islander mental health*. Vol. 1&2. Canberra: Australian Government Publishing Service.

Terr, L. (1990). *Too scared to cry: Psychic trauma in childhood*. New York: Harper & Row Publishers.

United Nations. (2008). *UN Declaration on the Rights of Indigenous Peoples*. United Nations. Retrieved from https://www.un.org/esa/socdev/unpfii/documents/faq_drips_en.pdf

Van der Kolk, B. (2007). Trauma and memory. *Encyclopedia of Stress* (pp. 765-767). doi:10.1016/b978-012373947-6.00381-0

Van der Kolk, B., & McFarlane. A. (1998). The black hole of trauma. In J. Rivkin & M. Ryan (Eds.), *Literary theory: An anthology* (pp. 487-502). Oxford: Blackwell Publishing Ltd.

Wilson, R. D., & Australian Human Rights and Equal Opportunity Commission. (1997). National Inquiry into the Separation of Aboriginal and Torres Strait Islander Children from their Families (Australia). *Bringing them home: Report of the National Inquiry into the Separation of Aboriginal and Torres Strait Islander Children from their Families*. Sydney: Human Rights and Equal Opportunity Commission.

World Health Organization. (2014). *Mental health: A state of well-being*. World Health Organization. Retrieved from: https://www.who.int/features/factfiles/mental_health/en/

CHAPTER NINE

The older person

Jessica Biles and Brett Biles

Warning: This chapter contains sensitive information related to death and dying that may cause distress to Aboriginal and Torres Strait Islander readers.

LEARNING CONCEPTS

Studying this chapter should enable you to:

1. identify the demographics of older Aboriginal and Torres Strait Islander people within Australia.
2. identify social and emotional perspectives of older Aboriginal and Torres Strait Islander people.
3. explore chronic and complex care in relation to older Aboriginal and Torres Strait Islander people.
4. explore the role of the carer in relation to older Aboriginal and Torres Strait Islander people.
5. explore foundational dementia care in relation to older Aboriginal and Torres Strait Islander people.
6. explore palliative care in the context of Aboriginal and Torres Strait Islander peoples' health and wellness, with a focus on the older person.

KEY TERMS

ageing well

carer

complex care

older Aboriginal and Torres Strait Islander people

Stolen Generations

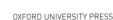

Introduction

This chapter will encourage you to begin thinking about the relevance of health perspectives related to older Aboriginal and Torres Strait Islander people.

older Aboriginal and Torres Strait Islander people Aboriginal and Torres Strait Islander people who are over 50 years of age.

The Australian Institute of Health and Welfare (2011) identifies **older Aboriginal and Torres Strait Islander people** as those people aged 50 and above. In Australia, this accounts for 12% of the Aboriginal and Torres Strait Islander population nationally (Australian Institute of Health and Welfare, 2015). Older non-Indigenous Australians are classified as 65 years and above, which is due to the health-related conditions that affect Aboriginal and Torres Strait Islander people at a younger age (Australian National Audit Office, 2017). Nationally, the Aboriginal and Torres Strait Islander population is projected to increase across all age groups, and by 2026 the number of people aged 55 and above is projected to more than double (a 114% increase) (Australian Institute of Health and Welfare, 2015), making Aboriginal and Torres Strait Islander people's aged care a priority focus area. As noted, the classification of the older person within Aboriginal and Torres Strait Islander communities begins earlier than for other Australians (Sivertsen, Harrington & Hamiduzzaman, 2018), requiring a considered approach in mainstream healthcare services.

Within Australia, 79% of Aboriginal and Torres Strait Islander people reside in non-remote areas (Australian Institute of Health and Welfare, 2011, 2018), emphasising not only the need for strategic thought in health service priority areas but also the importance of regional support services.

Social and emotional wellbeing

As previously identified in Chapter 3, health service delivery in Australia is not always aligned with the definition of health or the health needs of Aboriginal and Torres Strait Islander peoples (Farrelly & Lumby, 2008). This is a major concern for the care provided to Aboriginal and Torres Strait Islander peoples. Care needs to be person-specific and the health practitioner needs to be aware that the cultural beliefs from one nation may differ markedly from another (Browne & Varcoe, 2006). The diversity within Aboriginal and Torres Strait Islander communities influences the care provided, and nurses and allied health professionals need to be aware of cultural diversity not only between communities but also within communities and respond accordingly (Thackrah & Scott, 2010).

Within Aboriginal and Torres Strait Islander communities, the older person is respected, offers wisdom and is the cultural guide for younger generations (Thackrah & Scott, 2010). This is a major role and should be borne in mind by nurses and allied health professionals. With the majority of older people residing in regional locations (Australian Institute of Health and Welfare, 2018), the ability to access metropolitan-based care may be reduced. Given the extended and important role of older people within Aboriginal and Torres Strait Islander communities, care planning needs to be based on their individual needs and in consultation with the wider/extended family (Nash, Meiklejohn & Sacre, 2006).

As discussed in Chapter 2, the **Stolen Generations** are those people who were taken from their families as result of government policy in Australia (Wilson & Australian Human Rights and Equal Opportunity Commission, 1997). According to the *Bringing them Home* report, children were forcibly removed from their families by the Australian government well into the 1970s (Wilson & Australian Human Rights and Equal Opportunity Commission, 1997). The implications of this are wide, traumatic and varied. The reality for nursing and allied health professionals is that the implications remain real and raw for older peoples today.

Within older Aboriginal and Torres Strait Islander populations in 2018, almost 21,000 individuals were surviving members of the Stolen Generations (Australian Institute of Health and Welfare, 2018). 66% were aged over 50 years, while 20% were aged over 65 years with complex healthcare needs and in general poorer health (Australian Institute of Health and Welfare, 2018).

As noted above, within Aboriginal and Torres Strait Islander communities the older person holds the responsibility of the spiritual and cultural heritage, maintaining connection to country, caring for family (including grandchildren), and providing leadership and support within the community (LoGiudice, 2016; Smith et al., 2011). The World Health Organization's definition of **ageing well** is 'optimising opportunities for good health, so that older people can take an active part in society and enjoy an independent and high quality of life' (World Health Organization, 2015). The *National Aboriginal and Torres Strait Islander Health Plan 2013–2023* (Commonwealth of Australia, 2013, p. 40) states: 'Older Aboriginal and Torres Strait Islander people are able to live out their lives as active, healthy, culturally secure and comfortably as possible'.

The importance of older Aboriginal and Torres Strait Islander people is not to be underestimated or misunderstood. The connection to land and communities is interlinked and often results in increased pressure to remain on country (LoGiudice, 2016). This is important to nursing and allied health professionals for being able to understand the complexities of treatments for chronic and complex care requiring regional, rural and remote access for the older client, with the priority to ensure culturally competent services for the older client.

Chronic and complex care

Complex care should focus not only on the biomedical model of healthcare but also on the social, emotional and spiritual care needs of the older person (Johnson & Chang, 2014). This requires clinicians who are aware of the needs of older clients but most importantly health services that are responsive to the needs of the older client.

Stolen Generations
Those people who were taken away from their families as result of government policy in Australia (Wilson & Australian Human Rights and Equal Opportunity Commission, 1997).

ageing well 'Optimising opportunities for good health, so that older people can take an active part in society and enjoy an independent and high quality of life' (World Health Organization, 2015).

complex care Care that focuses on the social, emotional and spiritual care needs of the older person (Johnson & Chang, 2015).

Worldwide we see healthcare not delivering outcomes to vulnerable populations, which includes older people. Nurses and allied health professionals work in systems that at times resemble 'silos' that do not respond to the needs of the older person (Goodwin, 2015). The challenge for the modern-day health professional is how best to deliver in a system that doesn't provide integrated care. How to work beyond systems and look to the person largely remains a challenge for the future. Non-government organisations and community-based care become paramount when considering the complex needs of a client, as does the approach to care by the individual health professional (Australian Health Ministers' Advisory Council, 2017).

Within Australia we see five national health priority areas that link to complex care. Four of these priority areas—cardiovascular health, cancer control, mental health and diabetes mellitus—are relevant to older Aboriginal and Torres Strait Islander people (Australian Institute of Health and Welfare, 2018). Within the *National Aboriginal and Torres Strait Islander Health Plan 2013–2023* (Commonwealth of Australia, 2013), we discover that revised targets for older people relate to health checks and immunisations. The focus on these suggests that access to healthcare needs to be a priority, with health services being able to demonstrate a sense of culturally responsive care. These principles of culturally responsive care include adequate funding, 'proper' consultation, participation, leadership and quality assurance (LoGiudice, 2016), with the key focus being on enhancing resilience, empowerment and local workforce engagement to care for older Aboriginal and Torres Strait Islander people. Examples of this culturally responsive care include the Yuendumu Old People's Programme; Lungurra Ngoora, a pilot model of care in a remote Aboriginal community; and the Rumbalara Elders facility, a 30-bed residential-care home in Shepparton that includes independent living apartments, full-time care suites and a palliative care unit (Australian Indigenous HealthInfoNet, 2019).

The role of the carer

carer One who provides unpaid care and support to family and friends who have a disability, social and emotional wellbeing problems, chronic and complex conditions, or terminal illness (Carers Australia, 2018).

The **carer** provides unpaid care and support to family and friends who have a disability, social and emotional wellbeing problems, chronic and complex conditions, or a terminal illness (Carers Australia, 2018). Carers play an integral role in complex disease management, which can include physical and personal care (showering, feeding, dressing, lifting, transport, etc.), medication management, and emotional, social and financial support (Carers Australia, 2018). In 2015, there were 2.7 million unpaid carers in Australia; 12.4% of Aboriginal and Torres Strait Islander people are carers compared to 10.5% of non-Indigenous people (Australian Bureau of Statistics, 2016).

As discussed earlier in this chapter, 79% of Aboriginal and Torres Strait Islander people reside in non-remote areas, so it is important to understand that there are environmental, social and economic impacts of living in regional areas that affect carers (Carers Australia, 2018). These include social isolation and barriers that limit access to health and welfare services (poor transport, limited information and limited opportunities for education and literacy). It is fundamental that there is a functional and culturally responsive health service that caters for the needs of older Aboriginal and Torres Strait Islander people and their carers, no matter how remote the setting.

Case study 9.1: Nursing focus

Mary and John's story

Mary is a 55-year-old Aboriginal woman who is married to John, who is 60 years of age. Mary and John are legal guardians of their three grandchildren: Tony (aged 10 years), Isabella (12) and Lily (14). Over the last few years, John's health has slowly deteriorated to the stage where he is requiring more health and wellbeing support. This extra support is placing a large amount of pressure on Mary, as she is trying to care for and support John as well as their three grandchildren. Mary has noticed that her health is also starting to decline. Mary has presented to her local Aboriginal Medical Service (AMS) for her annual check-up. You are the nurse who is undertaking the health assessment. During the assessment, Mary tells you that she is finding it very difficult to get John to all his medical appointments, juggle the grandchildren's needs and look after all the home requirements. Mary also mentioned that she is feeling extremely fatigued, has lost some weight over the last six months and is feeling really overwhelmed. Mary makes the comment: 'Something has to give because it is getting too much. I am unsure what I can do about this situation'.

CRITICAL REFLECTION QUESTIONS

- What are your initial responses to the concerns Mary has raised?
- What does Mary require at this stage? How would you find this out?
- What support services may be available for Mary and her family?

Case study 9.2: Allied health focus

Mary and John's story continued

Mary has been referred to the local allied health clinic after her health assessment at the AMS. You are the allied health professional on duty. You have reviewed Mary's history and have noted that Mary is extremely unsure about

(Continued)

what services she may be able to access to make caring for John and their three grandchildren a bit easier.

CRITICAL REFLECTION QUESTIONS

- What are your initial responses to this situation?
- As an allied health professional, what do you do in this situation?
- What services do you think you can offer Mary, and why?

Dementia care

Dementia has been defined as an irreversible condition of the brain (Alzheimer's Australia, 2007). There are many differing types of dementia that impact not only those suffering but also their extended family and carers. Within Aboriginal and Torres Strait Islander communities we can note a higher risk and higher prevalence of the disease, as well as noting that it commences at a much younger age (Australian Institute of Health and Welfare, 2011). Men seem to be at higher risk, with chronic diseases such as cardiovascular disease, type 2 diabetes, depression and smoking all adding to higher prevalence. Coupled with the links between childhood stress and emotional health, the rates of dementia are currently four to five times higher in Aboriginal and Torres Strait Islander peoples than in non-Indigenous populations (Goldberg, Cox, Hoang & Baldock, 2018). The data also suggest dementia is occurring across the lifespan rather than being an older person's disease (Alzheimer's Australia, 2007).

Within Aboriginal and Torres Strait Islander communities, we see access to culturally appropriate care as a major barrier, suggesting the focus needs to be on workforce development. Home care service rates are significantly higher than for non-Indigenous populations, with less than 1% of Aboriginal and Torres Strait Islander people in permanent residential aged care (Australian National Audit Office, 2017). These data are profound and suggest that the majority of those suffering from dementia live in their homes. For nurses and allied health professions, this is an important point to consider for professional practice and practice recommendations.

Case study 9.3: Nursing focus

Roy's story

Roy is a 65-year-old man from the Eora nation. Roy and his wife Mabel have been married for over 30 years. They have five children and 15 grandchildren. Roy and Mabel have been active support people for their children and grandchildren.

Lately Roy has noticed a decline in Mabel's health. She seems unable to focus on tasks, often failing to remember daily routines, and generally appears to be uninterested in aspects of their life that normally are important to her. Mabel is now unable to remember the names of her grandchildren, which is upsetting for the family. Roy also keeps finding the ice cream in the kitchen cupboard. Roy is concerned so he has booked an individual appointment at the Aboriginal Medical Centre where you work as a registered nurse. Roy seems distressed during the appointment and indicates he needs some support.

CRITICAL REFLECTION QUESTIONS

- What are your initial responses to this situation?
- How will you approach support with Roy?
- How will you consider the wider family in your discussion with Roy?

Case study 9.4: Allied health focus

Roy's story continued

Roy has been referred by the registered nurse at the Aboriginal Health Service at which you consult one day per week. Roy's wife Mabel has recently been diagnosed with early-stage dementia. As an allied health professional, you have been asked to offer Roy and his wife Mabel support strategies for their home. Your initial consultation is at the medical service where you hope to develop a rapport and start a professional relationship with both Roy and Mabel. You come from a non-Indigenous background and have heard that Roy is a local Elder.

CRITICAL REFLECTION QUESTIONS

- What are your initial responses to this situation?
- How will you culturally prepare for this consultation?
- How will you approach providing support for both Roy and Mabel?
- How will you consider the wider family in your discussions with Roy?

Care for those diagnosed with dementia

This section will focus on the care and support for individuals who are diagnosed with dementia. It will focus on family-centred support that involves strategies for carers as well as those suffering from dementia.

Family-centred care and support available

Family-centred care is an approach to care that aims to provide health equality to consumers of healthcare (Wolff & Boyd, 2015). The principles surrounding family-centred care aim to empower people with choice and the autonomy to make health decisions that work well for them. It is acknowledged that this may involve the support for family and or close friends in decision-making processes that support strengths-based outcomes for the individual (Wolff & Boyd, 2015). As previously discussed, the role of the older person in Aboriginal and Torres Strait Islander communities is wide and varied. When a diagnosis of dementia is formally made within a community, the effects can be isolating and devastating for the entire community. Because the older person passes on cultural knowledge, the impact of a debilitating disease that targets memory is severe (Flicker & Holdsworth, 2014). Thus care management that is focused on the family and not only the individual is paramount for the health professional. Central to family-centred care is trust (Johnson & Chang, 2016), so establishing meaningful forms of communication prior to assessment is also paramount.

A number of resources may be useful to the client and or their family. The following is a list of current documents that may be useful in the provision of care:

- *Dementia Learning Resource for Aboriginal and Torres Strait Islander Communities*, 2nd edition (Alzheimer's Association (SA), Department of Health and Ageing & Ageing, Disability & Home Care (NSW), 2010)
- *Family, Friends and Community* booklet (Dementia Australia, 2016a)
- *The Fading Moon: A Dementia Resource for Aboriginal and Torres Strait Islander communities* [DVD] (Dementia Australia, 2016b)
- *Younger Onset Dementia* (Dementia Australia, 2018).

A focus on functional abilities and a strengths-based approach to care is paramount. Ensuring clients and families can access the support available can ease both the financial and emotional burden for newly diagnosed people. Within the Commonwealth, access to home support packages and the National Aboriginal and Torres Strait Islander Flexible Aged Care Program (NATSIFACP) is available (Australian National Audit Office, 2017). Local support can be found within specific communities, so it is fundamental that you get to know what services are available in your local and surrounding communities.

Assessment tools

Assessment tools are an important aspect to consider when responding to the needs of the older Aboriginal and Torres Strait Islander client with dementia. The Kimberley Indigenous Cognitive Assessment tool was developed in response to a demand for Aboriginal and Torres Strait Islander specific needs being identified in mainstream assessment tools (LoGiudice, Smith, Thomas, Lautenschlager, Almeida, Atkinson & Flicker, 2006). This tool has the capacity to be adapted to a variety of languages and identifies the importance of family-centred care and experiences that need to be considered by health professionals (Western Australian Centre for Health and Aging, 2004; Johnson & Chang, 2014). This has since been validated and redeveloped as the Indigenous Cognitive Assessment: KICA Assessment Tool Victoria for metropolitan and regional communities in Victoria (Johnson & Chang, 2014; LoGiudice, Gibson & Savvas, 2013).

In addition, community-based education is paramount. The *Dementia Learning Resource for Aboriginal and Torres Strait Islander Communities* (Alzheimer's Association (SA), Department of Health and Ageing & Ageing, Disability & Home Care (NSW), 2010) brings awareness and knowledge, and empowers communities in supporting and caring for those that have dementia.

Palliative care

Palliative Care Australia defines palliative care as 'person and family-centred care provided for a person with an active, progressive, advanced disease, who has little or no prospect of cure and who is expected to die, and for whom the primary treatment goal is to optimise the quality of life' (Palliative Care Australia, 2018, p. 5). Within Aboriginal and Torres Strait Islander communities, end-of-life care may be considered sacred and may have cultural traditions involved. Importantly, these traditions may not be widely known. Therefore, it is important when considering palliative care that consideration of potential traditions is provided by the health professionals (Aboriginal & Torres Strait Islander Health Branch, Queensland Health, 2015).

In 2017, only 1.4% of Aboriginal and Torres Strait Islander people had registered links with palliative care services. In addition, the rate of acute hospitalisations was twice that of non-Indigenous populations (Australian Institute of Health and Welfare, 2018). This suggests that home care support, care planning and equity in service delivery remains unresponsive to the needs of Aboriginal and Torres Strait Islander peoples, which provides a focus point for future research (Australian Institute of Health and Welfare, 2018). A need for cultural understanding seems an appropriate way forward. Interestingly, within Aboriginal and Torres Strait Islander communities hospitalisations often indicate the period of time where death is close (Aboriginal & Torres Strait Islander Health Branch, Queensland Health, 2015). Acute care health professionals should consider this when attending to holistic care.

During the decision-making processes around end-of-life care within Aboriginal and Torres Strait Islander communities, it is imperative that the client is asked who they wish to include in the decision making and whose support they would like in health-related meetings (Program of Experience in the Palliative Approach, 2014).

Decision making may be shared and may involve a number of people (Program of Experience in the Palliative Approach, 2014).

In a study conducted in the Northern Territory it was identified that seven principles are important to Aboriginal and Torres Strait Islander people in the final stages of life (McGrath & Holewa, 2006). These include but are not limited to the following: equity; autonomy/empowerment; trust; humane, non-judgmental care; seamless care; emphasis on living; and cultural respect. These fundamental aspects of care indicate the importance of health professional collaboration that is respectful, holistic and client-centred.

Recently, Palliative Care Australia has led the revision of the National Palliative Care Standards (2018), which mandate nine standards aimed at improving practice and quality of care. Most importantly, the standards mandate palliative care as everyone's business, with a drive towards ensuring empowered decision making by the client. The standards indicate compassionate and unbiased care as being paramount for all involved (Palliative Care Australia, 2018). It is evidenced that planned and coordinated care that is responsive to the needs of the client (emotional, spiritual, cultural and physical) will lead to a client-centred approach (Palliative Care Australia, 2011).

Case study 9.5: Nursing focus

Mary and John's story continued

After a period of significant illness, John has been diagnosed with end-stage lung cancer with metastatic liver cancer. Mary, John, Tony, Isabella and Lily are devastated by this diagnosis. After much consideration, John has decided to prepare for his end-of-life care. You are the nurse who is undertaking a consultation to commence conversations on John's advanced care plan.

CRITICAL REFLECTION QUESTIONS

- What are the nursing considerations relating to John's situation?
- How will you implement a family-centred care approach?
- What support services may be available for John, Mary, Tony, Isabella and Lily?

Case study 9.6: Allied health focus

Mary and John's story continued

Following John's diagnosis, he has been referred to you by the registered nurse. You are the team leader of a rural allied health team and would like to refer the family to available services. After reviewing the registered nurse's handover, you decide that an occupational therapist home visit is required, along with a physiotherapy mobility assessment. You schedule an initial meeting with John and his family.

CRITICAL REFLECTION QUESTIONS

- As the team leader, how would you implement a plan of care to ensure that John and his family are well informed?
- How will you ensure that you are responsive to John's palliative care plan?
- What services do you think you can offer Mary, and why?

Practical skills for health professionals

Each client is unique and will require different foci at differing stages of their disease. However, practical skills for health professionals can be incorporated into individual circumstances. This section will provide some practical skills that health professionals can embed in their day-to-day practice.

Diagnosis

Within Aboriginal and Torres Strait Islander communities, there may be a need to discuss the diagnosis and treatment with wider family members. Ensure that consultation times allow for this and that they are well documented to ensure the wishes of the client, family members and carers are well supported (Aboriginal & Torres Strait Islander Health Branch, Queensland Health, 2015). Be mindful of the role of older people within communities and ensure that you acknowledge and respond to diversity.

Trust

As discussed in previous chapters, mistrust of mainstream health systems is common within Aboriginal and Torres Strait Islander communities (Palliative Care Australia, 2018). Remember that when working as a health professional, you represent the system in which you are employed. Consider ways that you can demonstrate trust. For example, you may consider your terminology, body language, and approach to healthcare, as well as the notions of men's and women's business. Consider your own personal worldview and how this may influence the care opportunities that you provide.

Pain management

Acknowledging pain may be viewed as weakness within some Aboriginal and Torres Strait Islander peoples, meaning that pain relief may not be requested (Aboriginal & Torres Strait Islander Health Branch, Queensland Health, 2015). This requires the health professional to perform regular pain-management assessments to ensure the client is comfortable.

Returning to country

Returning to country is spiritually important for Aboriginal and Torres Strait Islander peoples before death (Aboriginal & Torres Strait Islander Health Branch, Queensland Health, 2015). This may present complexities if the client requires extensive therapy that is not available on country (Northern Sydney Local Health District, 2015). It is important for the health professional to acknowledge this situation. Liaising closely with smaller communities and accessing telehealth and community-based services may be useful options to explore.

Before death

As discussed, Elders play a significant role within a community. If a client is close to death and is an inpatient of a health service, it is important to ensure that the client is in a spacious room, as they may have a large volume of visitors paying their respects. Visiting hours also may need to be varied (Northern Sydney Local Health District, 2015).

Following death

Within some Aboriginal and Torres Strait Islander communities, the name of the deceased becomes taboo after they have died. It is also considered inappropriate for non-Indigenous people to contact next of kin to advise of the death (Aboriginal & Torres Strait Islander Health Branch, Queensland Health, 2015). Liaise closely with Aboriginal Health Workers and liaison officers during this time. Acknowledge diversity in Aboriginal and Torres Strait Islander nations and customs, and stay educated on sensitive matters and protocols (Palliative Care Australia, 2018).

Sorry business

Sorry business is an important tradition that acknowledges the death of a person while providing support to family and friends. It marks the start of the journey of the deceased spirit and is bound by many customs and traditions that are dependent on the nation of the deceased person (Palliative Care Australia, 2018). This time may involve large family gatherings and extended support, as well as formal traditions such as:

- not mentioning the deceased's name—mentioning the name is believed to result in the deceased person's spirit being called back from the next world, which is considered detrimental (Aboriginal & Torres Strait Islander Health Branch, Queensland Health, 2015)
- avoiding eye contact of the family members of the deceased as a mark of respect (Northern Sydney Local Health District, 2015)
- holding a smoking ceremony to encourage the spirit's descent into the next world (Aboriginal & Torres Strait Islander Health Branch, Queensland Health, 2015).

As health professionals it is important that we are respectful of traditions and protocols, enabling them to be expressed within mainstream health structures, and that we continue on a journey of Indigenous Australian cultural competence. It is not the responsibility of clients to inform us of their wishes but for us to maintain our own education and enable space in our practice for conversations to emerge.

Conclusion

Older Aboriginal and Torres Strait Islander people bring a unique perspective to health. This perspective is an area that nursing and allied health professionals need to understand to be able to identify individual requirements and acknowledge the importance of family-centred care. A collaborative approach to healthcare is absolutely fundamental to ensure older Aboriginal and Torres Strait Islander people are given the dignity and respect that is required and deserved. Older Aboriginal and Torres Strait Islander people hold the responsibility of the spiritual and cultural heritage, maintaining connection to country, caring for family (including grandchildren), and providing leadership and support within the community.

SUMMARY

This chapter has encouraged you to consider the role of the older Aboriginal and Torres Strait Islander person. It has encouraged you to consider cultural aspects of care that focus on the strength of each individual client.

Learning concept 1

Identify the demographics of older Aboriginal and Torres Strait Islander people within Australia: The Australian Institute of Health and Welfare (2011) identifies older Aboriginal and Torres Strait Islander people as those people aged 50 and above. In Australia this accounts for 12% of the Aboriginal and Torres Strait Islander population nationally.

Learning concept 2

Identify social and emotional perspectives of older Aboriginal and Torres Strait Islander people: Within Aboriginal and Torres Strait Islander communities, the older person is respected, offers wisdom and is the cultural guidance for younger generations (Thackarah & Scott, 2010). This is a major role and should be considered by nurses and allied health professionals in their dealings with community members.

Learning concept 3

Explore chronic and complex care in relation to older Aboriginal and Torres Strait Islander people: This requires clinicians who are aware not only of the needs of older clients but more importantly the health services that are responsive to the needs of the older client. Worldwide we see healthcare not delivering outcomes to vulnerable populations, which includes older people. Nurses and allied health professionals work in systems that at times resemble 'silos' that do not respond to the needs of the older person (Goodwin, 2015).

Learning concept 4

Explore the role of the carer in relation to older Aboriginal and Torres Strait Islander people: Carers provide unpaid care and support to family and friends who have a disability, social and emotional wellbeing problems, chronic and complex conditions or a terminal illness (Carers Australia, 2018). Carers play an integral role in complex disease management, which can include physical and personal care (showering, feeding, dressing, lifting, transport, etc.), medication management, and emotional, social and financial support (Carers Australia, 2018).

Learning concept 5

<u>Explore foundational dementia care in relation to older Aboriginal and Torres Strait Islander people:</u> Within Aboriginal and Torres Strait Islander communities, there is a higher risk and higher prevalence of the disease, and it commences at a much younger age (Australian Institute of Health and Welfare, 2011). Family-centred care is an approach to care that aims to provide health equality to consumers of healthcare (Wolff & Boyd, 2015). The principles surrounding family-centred care are around empowering people with choice and providing them with the autonomy to make health decisions that work well for them. It is acknowledged that this may involve the support of family and/or close friends in decision-making processes that support strengths-based outcomes for the individual (Wolff & Boyd, 2015).

Learning concept 6

<u>Explore palliative care in the context of Aboriginal and Torres Strait Islander peoples' health and wellness, with a focus on the older person:</u> Within Aboriginal and Torres Strait Islander communities, end-of-life care may be considered sacred and may have cultural traditions involved. Importantly, these traditions may not be widely known. Therefore, it is important when considering palliative care that consideration of potential traditions is provided by the health professionals.

REVISION QUESTIONS

1. Why is the older person in Aboriginal and Torres Strait Islander communities so important?
2. What role does the older Aboriginal and Torres Strait Islander person play in the community?
3. Critique this chapter and identify five practices that you will commit to implementing in your future practice.
4. Explore the concept of family-based care in relation to older Aboriginal and Torres Strait Islander people.

FURTHER READINGS/ADDITIONAL RESOURCES

Carers Australia. (2018). *Resources for Aboriginal and Torres Strait Islander carers*. Retrieved from http://www.carersaustralia.com.au/about-carers/aboriginalandtorresstraitislandercarers/resources-for-aboriginal-and-torres-strait-islander-carers2/

REFERENCES

Aboriginal & Torres Strait Islander Health Branch, Queensland Health. (2015). *Sad news, sorry business: Guidelines for caring for Aboriginal and Torres Strait Islander people through death and dying.* Brisbane: Queensland Health.

Alzheimer's Association (SA), Department of Health and Ageing & Ageing, Disability & Home Care (NSW). (2010). *Dementia learning resource for Aboriginal and Torres Strait Islander communities* (Version 2). Sydney: Ageing, Disability & Home Care (NSW).

Alzheimer's Australia. (2007). *Dementia: A major health problem for indigenous people.* Retrieved from https://www.dementia.org.au/files/20070800_Nat_NP_12DemMajHlthProbIndig.pdf

Australian Bureau of Statistics. (2016). *Disability, Ageing and Carers, Australia: Summary of findings, 2015.* ABS Cat. No. 4430.0. Canberra: ABS

Australian Health Ministers' Advisory Council. (2017). *Aboriginal and Torres Strait Islander Health Performance Framework 2017 Report.* Canberra: AHMAC.

Australian Indigenous HealthInfoNet. (2019). *Promote and practice—Programs.* Retrieved from https://healthinfonet.ecu.edu.au/key-resources/programs-and-projects

Australian Institute of Health and Welfare. (2011). *Older Aboriginal and Torres Strait Islander people.* https://www.aihw.gov.au/reports/indigenous-australians/older-aboriginal-and-torres-strait-islander-people/formats

Australian Institute of Health and Welfare. (2015). *The health and welfare of Australia's Aboriginal and Torres Strait Islander peoples 2015.* Cat. No. IHW 147. Canberra: AIHW.

Australian Institute of Health and Welfare. (2018). *Palliative care services in Australia.* Retrieved from https://www.aihw.gov.au/reports/palliative-care-services/palliative-care-services-in-australia/contents/summary

Australian National Audit Office. (2017). *Indigenous Aged Care. Performance Audit.* ANAO Report No. 53 2016–17. Retrieved from https://www.anao.gov.au/work/performance-audit/indigenous-aged-care

Browne, A., & Varcoe, C. (2006). Critical cultural perspectives and health care involving Aboriginal peoples. *Contemporary Nurse, 22*(2), 155-168. doi:10.5172/conu.2006.22.2.155

Carers Australia. (2018). *About carers.* Retrieved from http://www.carersaustralia.com.au/about-carers

Commonwealth of Australia. (2013). *National Aboriginal and Torres Strait Islander health plan 2013–2023.* Canberra: Commonwealth of Australia.

Dementia Australia. (2016a). *Aboriginal and Torres Strait Islander communities.* Retrieved from https://www.dementia.org.au/resources/for-aboriginal-and-torres-strait-islander-communities

Dementia Australia. (2016b). *The Fading Moon: A dementia resource for Aboriginal and Torres Strait Islander communities.* Retrieved from https://www.dementia.org.au/about-dementia/resources/videos/collections?playlist=Aboriginal%20and%20Torres%20Strait%20Islander

Dementia Australia. (2018). *Younger onset dementia.* Retrieved from https://www.dementia.org.au/files/resources/2018-Dementia-Australia-ATSI-YOD-Keyworker-Brochure.pdf

Farrelly, T., & Lumby, B. (2008). Aboriginal ageing and disability issues in south west and inner west Sydney. *Aboriginal and Islander Health Worker Journal*, 32(5), 27-34. Retrieved from https://search.informit.com.au/documentSummary;dn=328288041621257;res=IELHEA

Flicker, L., & Holdsworth, K. (2014). Aboriginal and Torres Strait Islander people and dementia: A review of the research. *Alzheimer's Australia Paper*, 41, 15-16. Retrieved from https://www.dementia.org.au/files/Alzheimers_Australia_Numbered_Publication_41.pdf

Goldberg, L. R., Cox, T., Hoang, H., & Baldock, D. (2018). Addressing dementia with Indigenous peoples: A contributing initiative from the Circular Head Aboriginal community [Letter]. *Australian and New Zealand Journal of Public Health*, 42(5), 424-426. Retrieved from https://doi.org/10.1111/1753-6405.12798.

Goodwin, N. (2015). How should integrated care address the challenge of people with complex health and social care needs? Emerging lessons from international case studies. *International Journal of Integrated Care*, 15(3). doi: http://doi.org/10.5334/ijic.2254

Johnson, A., & Chang, E. (2014). *Caring for older persons in Australia: Principles for nursing practice.* Milton: Wiley & Sons.

LoGiudice, D. (2016). The health of older Aboriginal and Torres Strait Islander peoples. *Australasian Journal on Ageing Early*, 35(2), 82-85.

LoGiudice, D., Gibson, S., Savvas, S. (2013). *Indigenous Cognitive Assessment—Modification and validation of the KICA in Victoria. Phase 1.* Australia: National Ageing Research Institute.

LoGiudice, D., Smith, K., Thomas, J., Lautenschlager, N. T., Almeida, O. P., Atkinson, D., & Flicker, L. (2006). Kimberley Indigenous Cognitive Assessment tool (KICA): Development of a cognitive assessment tool for older Indigenous Australians. *International Psychogeriatrics*, 18(2), 269-280.

McGrath, P., & Holewa, H. (2006). Seven principles for Indigenous palliative care service delivery: Research findings from Australia. *Austral-Asian Journal of Cancer*, 5(3), 179-186.

Nash. R., Meiklejohn. B., & Sacre. S. (2006). The Yapunyah project: Embedding Aboriginal and Torres Strait Islander perspectives in the nursing curriculum, *Contemporary Nurse*, 22(2), 296-316. doi: 10.5172/conu.2006.22.2.296

Northern Sydney Local Health District. (2015). *Death and dying in Aboriginal and Torres Strait Islander culture (sorry business). A framework for supporting Aboriginal and Torres Strait Islander peoples through sad news and sorry business.* Retrieved from https://www.nslhd.health.nsw.gov.au/Services/Directory/Documents/Death%20and%20Dying%20in%20Aboriginal%20and%20Torres%20Strait%20Islander%20Culture_Sorry%20Business.pdf

Palliative Care Australia. (2011). *Improving access to quality care at the end of life for Aboriginal and Torres Strait Islander Australians Position Statement.* Available at http://palliativecare.org.au/wp-content/uploads/2015/08/ PCA-Palliative-care-and-Indigenous-Australians-positionstatement-updated-16-8-11.pdf, accessed 19/12/2017

Palliative Care Australia. (2018). *National palliative care standards* (5th ed.). Canberra: Palliative Care Australia.

Program of Experience in the Palliative Approach. (2014). *Cultural considerations: Providing end of life care for Aboriginal peoples and Torres Strait Islander peoples* (pp. 32). Canberra: Author.

Sivertsen, N., Harrington, A., & Hamiduzzaman, M. (2018). The importance of integrating cultural and spiritual care into Aboriginal aged care. *Australian Nursing and Midwifery Journal*, 25(7), 39. Retrieved from https://search.informit.com.au/documentSummary;dn=354168275711328;res=IELHEA

Smith, K., Flicker, L., Shadforth, G., Carroll, E., Ralph, N., Atkinson, D., ... LoGiudice, D. (2011). 'Gotta be sit down and worked out together': Views of Aboriginal caregivers and service providers on ways to improve dementia care for Aboriginal Australians. *Rural and Remote Health*, 11(2), 1650.

Thackrah, R., & Scott, K. (2010). *Indigenous Australian health and cultures: An introduction for health professionals*. Perth: Pearson Australia

Western Australian Centre for Health and Aging. (2004). *Urban modified Kimberley Indigenous Cognitive Assessment*. Retrieved from https://www.perkins.org.au/wacha/our-research/indigenous/kica/

Wilson, R. D., & Australian Human Rights and Equal Opportunity Commission. (1997). *Bringing them home: National Inquiry into the Separation of Aboriginal and Torres Strait Islander Children from their Families.* Sydney: Human Rights and Equal Opportunity Commission.

Wolff, J. L., & Boyd, C. M. (2015). A Look at person-centered and family-centered care among older adults: Results from a national survey. *Journal of General Internal Medicine*, 30(10), 1497-1504. doi:10.1007/s11606-015-3359-6

World Health Organization. (2015). *World report on ageing and health 2015*. Retrieved from http://www.who.int/ageing/events/world-report-2015-launch/en/

GLOSSARY

Aboriginal Community Controlled Health Service (ACCHS)

A primary healthcare service initiated and operated by a local Aboriginal community to deliver holistic, comprehensive and culturally appropriate healthcare to the community, which controls it through a locally elected board made up of Aboriginal people.

ageing well

'Optimising opportunities for good health, so that older people can take an active part in society and enjoy an independent and high quality of life' (World Health Organization, 2015).

allied health professionals

A broad range of healthcare providers—other than doctors, nurses and dentists—who work as part of the multi-disciplinary team to provide and support the delivery of person-centred care.

burden of disease

A global standard for the assessment and comparison of the impact of different diseases, conditions or injuries on a specific population.

cardiac rehabilitation (CR)

A program where those with cardiac disease, their family and carers are supported by health professionals.

cardiovascular disease (CVD)

The term used to describe all conditions and diseases that affect the heart and blood vessels.

carer

One who provides unpaid care and support to family and friends who have a disability, social and emotional wellbeing problems, chronic and complex conditions, or terminal illness (Carers Australia, 2018).

community

A group of people living in the same place, sharing and having similar interests and attitudes in common.

complex care

Care that focuses on the social, emotional and spiritual care needs of the older person (Johnson & Chang, 2015).

critical reflection

A deep form of reflective learning that creates the opportunity for our worldviews to be transformed.

culture

A set of common beliefs, attitudes and norms shared by a group.

Dadirri

Deep listening, observing and maintaining relationships with others.

empowerment

The ability to take control of daily challenges without feeling overwhelmed.

endocrine disorder

A condition affecting the body and its function due to alteration in the secretion of, or body response to, a hormone.

Ethnocentrism

The lens through which one views the world being dominated by a reflection of people's perceptions (Matsumoto & Juang, 2004).

Fifth National Mental Health and Suicide Prevention Plan 2017

A commitment from all governments to work together to achieve integrated planning and service delivery of mental health and suicide prevention related services. It commits to a nationally agreed set of priority areas and actions to achieve an integrated mental health system that is stronger, more transparent, accountable, efficient and effective.

Gayaa Dhuwi (Proud Spirit) Declaration 2015

A commitment to improve the mental health of Aboriginal and Torres Strait Islander peoples. The name of the declaration was coined from 'Gayaa', which means happy, pleased and proud, and 'Dhuwi', which means 'spirit' in the Yuwaalaraay and Gamilaraay languages of northwest New South Wales.

health literacy

Personal skills, knowledge, motivation and capacity to access, understand and use information to make decisions about one's health and healthcare choices.

history

Not a series of agreed facts but something open to interpretation and argument; the telling of history itself changes over time as we ask new questions about the past.

holistic

The idea that parts of a whole are interconnected and interdependent.

Indigenous Australian cultural competence

A nonlinear process in which non-Indigenous health workers consider how their values, beliefs and behaviour influence the care they provide to Aboriginal and Torres Strait Islander peoples.

Indigenous concept of social and emotional wellbeing

Connects the health of Aboriginal and Torres Strait Islander peoples to the health of their family, kin and community, and their connection to country, culture, spirituality and ancestry (Calma, Dudgeon & Bray, 2017).

Indigenous health

'Not just the physical well-being of the individual but the social, emotional and cultural well-being of the whole community in which each individual is able to achieve their full potential as a human being, thereby bringing about the total wellbeing of their Community' (National Aboriginal Health and Strategy Working Party, 1989, p. x).

interprofessional collaboration

Where two or more professional groups work together towards client-centred goals.

mental health

'A state of wellbeing in which every individual realises his or her own potential, can cope with the normal stresses of life, can work productively and fruitfully, and is able to make a contribution to her or his community' (World Health Organization, 2014).

metabolic syndrome

A cluster of risk factors that results from an interplay of physiological, biochemical, clinical and metabolic factors, which results in a person presenting with hyperlipidaemia, hypertension and type 2 diabetes simultaneously.

methodology

A system of methods used in a particular discipline or area of activity.

National Strategic Framework for Aboriginal and Torres Strait Islander Peoples' Mental Health and Social and Emotional Wellbeing 2017–2023

A framework dedicated to Aboriginal and Torres Strait Islander peoples' social and emotional wellbeing and mental health. It is a stepped care guide aimed at supporting policy and practice.

older Aboriginal and Torres Strait Islander people

Aboriginal and Torres Strait Islander people who are over 50 years of age.

perinatal period

The time of conception through to 12 months after a baby is born.

primary healthcare

A philosophy of care based on social justice and an organising framework guiding health professionals to facilitate equitable social environments, equal access to healthcare and community and client empowerment through public participation (McMurray & Clendon, 2015).

privilege

A special right, advantage or immunity granted or available only to a particular person or group.

race

People identified as members of a group because of their physical appearance, culture or ethnic origin—real or supposed; the judgments made according to the presumed characteristics of that group.

racism

Prejudice, discrimination or antagonism directed against someone of a different race based on the belief that one's own race is superior.

reciprocity

A practice of exchange that yields mutual benefits.

social and emotional wellbeing

A term used to describe the social, emotional, spiritual and cultural wellbeing of a person. It recognises that connection to land, culture, spirituality, family and community is important to people and can influence their wellbeing. It also recognises that a person's social and emotional wellbeing is influenced by past and current policies and events.

social determinants of health
Interrelated social factors that determine health and wellbeing.

Stolen Generations
Those people who were taken away from their families as result of government policy in Australia (Wilson & Australian Human Rights and Equal Opportunity Commission, 1997).

suicide prevention
A commitment to reduce the risk of an individual taking their own life. It is arguable that it is not possible to entirely eliminate suicide, but it is possible to reduce the risk of it occurring.

transcultural care
Knowledge, skills and behaviours that are responsive to the delivery of healthcare to more than one culture.

United Nations Declaration on the Rights of Indigenous Peoples
A framework of minimum standards for the survival, dignity, wellbeing and rights of the world's indigenous peoples, including individual and collective rights; cultural rights and identity; rights to education, health, employment, language; and the right to remain separate and to pursue their own priorities in economic, social and cultural advance.

worldview
How we see, are and react to the world around us.

yarning
A term used by Aboriginal and Torres Strait Islander people to mean a conversation or dialogue between Aboriginal and Torres Strait Islander people.

INDEX

OXFORD UNIVERSITY PRESS